Discharged but came up as

27 FEB 83

17 DEC 92
21 JAN 92
9 FEB 92

THE Arthritis HELPBOOK

What you can do for your arthritis

Kate Lorig, R.N., Dr.P.H.

HEALTH EDUCATOR
STANFORD ARTHRITIS CENTER

James F. Fries, M.D.

ASSOCIATE PROFESSOR OF MEDICINE
STANFORD UNIVERSITY SCHOOL OF MEDICINE

CONTRIBUTING AUTHORS

DEBORAH STINCHFIELD, R.P.T.   *Physical Therapist*
INGRID SAUSJORD MOORE, R.D., M.P.H.   *Nutritionist*
SHARONA SILVERMAN, M.P.H.   *Health Educator*
DORIS MEYER, O.T.R.   *Occupational Therapist*
BARBARATERRY KURTZ, M.S.W., M.P.H.   *Social Worker*

GRAPHICS   SHARON LEIBOLT HATHAWAY

UK Edition revised and edited by
J. H. K. Reeves, M.D.

SOUVENIR PRESS

First published in the U.S.A. by
Addison-Wesley Publishing Company

First British Edition published 1983 by
Souvenir Press Ltd., 43 Great Russell Street London WC1B 3PA

ISBN 0 285 62574 8

Printed in Great Britain by
Hazell Watson & Viney Ltd,
Aylesbury, Bucks

To our 300 group leaders
and to over 4000
Arthritis Self-Management class participants

ACKNOWLEDGMENTS

We would like especially to thank the Stanford Arthritis Center folks: Pat Spitz, Gene Fauro Pratt, Dee Simpson, Beth Kant, Audrey Schomer, R. Guy Kraines, Jim Standish, Alison Harlow, Cathy Williams, Dr. Dennis McShane, Dr. Jeffrey Brown, Dr. Cody Wasner, Dr. Paul Feigenbaum, Dr. Halsted Holman, Dr. Andrei Calin, Dr. Melvin Britton, Dr. Tom Okarma, Dr. William Lages, and Dr. David Schurman. The Midpeninsula Health Service people: Dr. Joseph Hopkins, Judy Staples, Debbie Ridley, Joan Willingham, Jeanne Ewy, Dori Smith, Mary Ann Goodrich, Luann Ciccone, Virginia de Lemos, Sally Semans, and Sarah Reese. The U.C. Berkeley Health Education faculty: Dr. Robert Miller, Dr. Andrew Fisher, Dr. William Griffiths, Dr. Meredith Minkler, Dr. Carol D'Onofrio, and Dr. John Ratcliffe. Significant others: Dr. Robert Swezey, John Staples, Donna Holsted, Carol Rice, Jane Dito, Marie Cascio, Bea Mandel, Dr. Lawrence Green, Dr. Sarah Archer, Janice Pigg, and Carol Simpson. Bonnie Obrig and Sharon Joseph performed yeoman service in manuscript preparation, while Scip Wylbur typed and retyped tirelessly. To all of these fine people our deepest appreciation.

CONTENTS

PREFACE

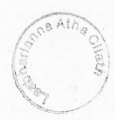

Before we start we would like to say a little about how this book came to be written and what we have learned in the process.

In 1979 the Stanford Arthritis Center began giving lessons to persons with arthritis. (From the very beginning our class members told us that they did not want to be called "patients.") The classes were taught by 40 people from our community who have arthritis or who are interested in arthritis. With a few exceptions, the teachers were not health professionals. The Arthritis Center staff worked with the teachers, and the lay teachers led the classes.

Our arthritis education classes use the same principles that we have presented earlier in *Take Care of Yourself, Taking Care of Your Child,* and *Arthritis. A Comprehensive Guide,* and they have benefited greatly from the many thousands of encouraging letters and helpful suggestions we have received. In these classes we are not concerned solely with improving knowledge. We also seek to help persons with arthritis change their activities and abilities, decrease their pain, and develop more confidence in themselves as caretakers for their bodies.

In our classes we emphasize three concepts:

1. Each person with arthritis is different. There is no one treatment that is right for everyone.

2. There are a number of things people can do to feel better. These things will not cure most kinds of arthritis, but they will help to relieve pain, maintain or increase mobility, and prevent deformity.

3. With knowledge, each individual is the best judge of which self-management techniques are best for him or her.

Therefore, this book was developed to give details about a variety of self-management treatments. We felt that it was not enough just to know that you should exercise. Instead, you must know about particular exercises, types of exercise, when to exercise, and how much to exercise. You need to understand the relationship between exercise and pain. The same considerations hold for what you need to know about relaxation, nutrition, joint protection, and all other self-management techniques. In *Arthritis. A Comprehensive Guide* we provided all the factual knowledge about arthritis. In this companion volume we try to help you use the information. This is a how-to-do-it book that has been developed with the help of many people very much like you.

When our class members first used this book they liked it but were quick to point out its faults: a neck exercise that caused too much pain, a nutrition section that was unclear, omission of a section on sleep disturbances, and so forth. Taking these suggestions we have added, revised, clarified, re-used, re-revised in a continuing cycle that has resulted in this present edition.

While only seven names appear on the title page as authors and contributors, this book was really written and guided by you, people with arthritis. As of late 1982, more than 4000 people have attended these classes and used this book. From all of them we have gained insights that we hope will be helpful to you.

All these people helped us in other ways, too. We have been carefully studying the effect of our classes on the way that people get along with their arthritis, and our class members have served as the subjects for these studies. In effect we "drew straws" to see which of the subjects on the waiting list would attend the next set of classes and which would have to wait four months. Then we compared how the people who went to the classes did with how the people on the waiting list did. Data from long questionnaires went into the computer, and after elaborate analyses we found what we had suspected all along.

People who exercise regularly (three to seven times a week), practice relaxation, and/or use any of the other self-management techniques have less pain and are more active than those people who are not arthritis self-managers. In addition, these people report that they go to the doctor less often (one and a-half visits less a year). These are the first controlled studies that have ever been done relating education programs in arthritis to outcomes, and they are very encouraging. The bottom line is that arthritis self-managers feel better! We would like to help you become an arthritis self-manager.

Now a few words of caution. First, you did not get stiff, painful joints overnight. Therefore, relief will not come quickly. Self-management is in no way a quick cure; it is a way of life to be practiced every day for the rest of your life. However, it is never too late to start. Our oldest self-manager was 96 when she first came to class.

Second, not everything works for everyone. Experiment, but give each activity two weeks to a month for first results. Don't give up too soon. If one thing does not work for you, try another.

Finally, this book is not meant to replace medical care. Rather, it is a supplement to that care. Most doctors do not have or do not take the time to explain exercises or joint protection in enough detail to help you very much. Therefore, we are hopeful that this book will assist both you and your physician. All of the advice and activities that we describe have been reviewed by many, many doctors, physical therapists, occupational therapists, nutritionists, and nurses, including the entire staff of the Stanford Arthritis Center. They represent a sound program essentially the same as that recommended by most health authorities today. If you have particular questions please talk them over with your doctor.

We would like you to feel that you are part of our cast of thousands. If you have comments or suggestions please send them to us by writing:

Stanford Arthritis Center
701 Welch Road, Suite 2208
Palo Alto, California 94304

Your suggestions will be reviewed and considered for our next edition. To all of you who helped in the past and who we couldn't name, many thanks, and to those of you who are just joining, a hearty welcome.

Stanford, California   K. L.

August 1982   J. F. F.

1
Arthritis
WHAT IS IT?

Arthritis. The very word evokes a spectre of fear and pain. People think of getting old, being unable to get around, and of becoming more dependent upon others. More so than with any other disease, the term "arthritis" carries with it a sense of hopelessness and futility. But the very opposite should be true. All arthritis can be helped.

In order to understand how to work with your arthritis, it is necessary to know a little about it. In fact, arthritis is not just a single disease. There are over 100 kinds of arthritis, all of which have something to do with one or more joints in the body. Even the word *arthritis* is misleading. The *arth* part comes from the Greek word meaning "joint," while *itis* means "inflammation or infection." Thus the word *arthritis* means "inflammation of the joint." The problem is that in many kinds of arthritis, the joint is not inflamed. A better description might be "problems with the joint."

The next step is to understand what a joint looks like and what the various parts do.

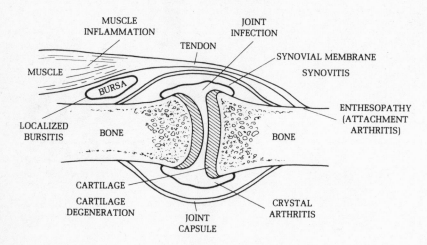

WHERE ARTHRITIS ATTACKS

A joint is a meeting of two bones for the purpose of allowing movement. It has the following six parts.

1. **Cartilage.** The end of each bone is covered with cartilage, a tough material that cushions and protects the ends of the bone. To get some idea of what cartilage is like, feel the middle of your nose or your ears. These are also made of cartilage. Cartilage in meat is "gristle."

2. **Synovial membrane (synovial sac).** Around each joint is the synovial sac, which protects the joint and also secretes the synovial fluid, which oils the joint. In fact, this fluid has many times the lubricating power of oil.

3. **Bursa.** A bursa is a small sac that is not part of the joint but is near the joint. It contains a fluid that lubricates the movement of muscles: muscle across muscle and muscle across bones. In some ways it is similar to the synovial sac.

4. **Muscle.** The muscles are elastic tissues that, by becoming shorter and longer, move the bones and thus move you.

5. **Tendon.** The tendons are fibrous cords that attach the muscles to the bones. You can feel them on the back of your hand or in the back of your knee.

6. **Ligament.** The ligaments are much shorter fibrous cords that attach bone to bone and reinforce the joint capsules.

When someone says, "I have arthritis," it means that something is wrong with one or more of these parts. For example, when the synovial membrane becomes inflamed, this is true arthritis. That is, the joint is inflamed. However, if the muscle becomes stretched from overexercise or is injured, this is not arthritis. The joint itself is not affected.

While there are over 100 types of arthritis, we will discuss only two major types—rheumatoid arthritis and osteoarthritis. If you are interested in knowing more about other types of arthritis, read *Arthritis. A Comprehensive Guide,* by Dr. James F. Fries (Reading, Mass.: Addison-Wesley, 1979).

2
Rheumatoid Arthritis
INFLAMED JOINTS

Rheumatoid arthritis (RA) is more than just arthritis. Indeed, many doctors call it "rheumatoid disease" to emphasize its widespread nature. The name is trying awkwardly to say the same thing; the term *rheum* refers to the stiffness, body aching, and fatigue that often accompany rheumatoid arthritis. Persons with RA often describe feeling much like they have a virus, with fatigue and aching in the muscles, except that, unlike a usual viral illness, the condition may persist for months or even years.

Three people out of every hundred get rheumatoid arthritis, amounting to approximately 1,500,000 people in Great Britain. Most of these people (about three-quarters) are women. The condition usually appears in middle life, in the forties or fifties, although it can begin at any age. Rheumatoid arthritis in children is quite different. Rheumatoid arthritis has been medically identified for about 200 years, although bone changes in the skeletons of some Mexican Indian groups suggest that the disease may have been around for thousands of years.

Since RA is so common, and because it can sometimes be severe, it is a major national health problem. It can result in difficulties with employment, problems with daily activities, and can put a severe stress on family relationships. In its most severe forms, and without good treatment, it can result in deformities of the joints. Fortunately, most people with RA do well and lead normal lives. Fear of rheumatoid arthritis, sometimes greatly exaggerated, can be as harmful as the disease itself.

In RA, the synovial membrane lining in the joint becomes inflamed. We don't have a good explanation as to why this inflammation starts, but the cells in the membrane divide and grow, and inflammatory cells come into the joint. Because of the bulk of these inflammatory cells, the joint become swollen, and feels puffy or boggy to the touch. The increased blood flow that is a feature of the inflammation makes the joint warm. The cells release chemicals (called *enzymes*) into the joint space and the enzymes cause further irritation and pain. If the process continues for years, the enzymes may gradually digest the cartilage and bone of the joint, actually eating away parts of the bone.

This then is rheumatoid arthritis, a process in which inflammation of the joint membrane, over many years, can cause damage to the joint itself.

FEATURES

Swelling and pain in one or more joints, lasting at least six weeks, are required for a diagnosis of rheumatoid arthritis. Usually, both sides of the body are affected similarly, and the arthritis is said to be "symmetrical." Often there are slight differences between the two sides, usually the right side being slightly worse in right-handed people and vice versa. Occasionally the condition skips about in an erratic fashion. The wrists and knuckles are almost always involved. The knees and the joints of the ball of the foot are often involved as well, and any joint can be affected. Of the knuckles, those at the base of the fingers are most frequently painful, while the joints at the ends of the fingers are often normal.

Lumps, usually between the size of a pea and a mothball, may form beneath the skin. These *rheumatoid nodules* are most commonly located near the elbow at the place where you rest your arms on the table, but they can pop up anywhere. Each represents an inflammation of a small blood vessel. They come and go during the course of the illness and usually are not a big problem. They do tend to occur in people with the most severe kinds of RA. Rarely, they become sore or infected, particularly if they are located around the ankle. Even more rarely, they form in the lungs or elsewhere in the body.

Laboratory tests sometimes can help a doctor recognize rheumatoid arthritis. The *rheumatoid factor* or *latex fixation* is the most commonly used blood test. Although this test may be negative in the first several months, it is eventually positive in about 80 percent of persons with RA. The rheumatoid factor is actually an antibody to certain body proteins and can sometimes be found in individuals with other diseases. Some doctors think that it is a way the body fights the disease, others think that it may play a role in causing the joint damage.

The ESR, which is short for *erythrocyte sedimentation rate*, is another frequently used test. It doesn't help in diagnosis, but it does help tell the severity of the disease. A high ESR (over 30 or so) suggests that the disease is quite active. The joint fluid is sometimes examined in rheumatoid arthritis in order to look at the inflammatory cells or to make sure that the joint is not infected with bacteria.

X-rays are not very helpful in the initial diagnosis of rheumatoid arthritis. It is unusual for changes to be seen in the bones or cartilage in the first few months of the disease, even when it is most severe. X-rays can help the doctor determine if damage to the bones or cartilage has occurred as the disease progresses. Some doctors like to get baseline X-rays to compare with later X-rays; we prefer to minimize the total number of X-rays.

Most people with RA notice problems in parts of their body other than the joints themselves. Usually, these are general problems such as muscle aches, fatigue, muscle stiffness (particularly in the morning), and even a low fever. Morning stiffness is often considered a hallmark of RA. After a rest period or even after just sitting motionless for a few minutes, the whole body feels stiff and is difficult to move. After a period of loosening up, motion becomes easier and less painful. People often have problems with fluid accumulation, particularly around the ankles. Occasionally, the rheumatoid disease may attack other body tissues, including the whites of the eyes, the nerves, the small arteries, and the lungs. Anaemia (low red blood cell count) is quite common, although it is seldom severe enough to need any treatment.

There can be unusual features due to the inflammation of the joint membrane. A *Baker's cyst* can form behind the knees and may feel like a tumour. It is just the synovial sac full of fluid, but it can extend down into the back of the calf and may cause pain.

Rheumatoid arthritis is one of the most complicated and mysterious diseases known. It is a challenge to patient and physician alike. Fortunately, the course of RA can be dramatically changed in most individuals. More so than with any other form of arthritis, if you have RA you need to develop an effective partnership with your doctor, as discussed in Chapter 13.

PROGNOSIS (THE FUTURE OF THE DISEASE)

Rheumatoid arthritis is the condition that most people think of when they hear the word *arthritis*. An image that comes to mind is of a person in a wheelchair, with swollen knees and twisted hands. True, most such people have rheumatoid arthritis. On balance, rheumatoid arthritis is the most destructive kind of arthritis known. Erosion of the bone itself, rupture of tendons, and slippage of the joints can result in crippling. But most people with rheumatoid arthritis do very, very much better than this. In fact, only one in six persons with RA develops any crippling or deformities at all. And it is probable that these could have been prevented by good, early treatment.

Rheumatoid arthritis varies greatly in severity and duration. Most favourable is the so-called "palindromic" rheumatism, where a brief illness lasting, at most, some months, is followed by complete resolution and no disability results. Many cases are mild and require no hospital treatment. The majority, about 65 per cent, have a course in which the disease fluctuates between exacerbations and remissions. At times the joints are "hot" and painful and this can be monitored by the ESR and other tests. A small proportion start with an acute flare up, are quite ill and need long hospitalization for rest and intensive treatment.

Whichever course the disease follows, severe disability and crippling only affects a small proportion of sufferers. Initially it is not possible to be certain what the prognosis is but if the blood test is positive for rheumatoid factor or the disease process is active for a year or more, it is likely that chronic rheumatism will follow.

Often it is hard for persons with RA and their relatives to appreciate that even the worst forms of rheumatoid arthritis tend to get better with time. The arthritis usually becomes less aggressive. The inflammation (synovitis) is less active and the fatigue and stiffness decrease. New joints are not likely to become involved after several years of disease. But even though the disease is less violent, any destruction of bones and ligaments that occurred in earlier years will persist. Thus deformities usually will not improve, even though no new damage is occurring. Hence, it is important to treat the disease correctly in the early years so that the joints will work well after the disease activity subsides.

TREATMENT

Treatment programmes for rheumatoid arthritis are often complicated and can be very confusing. In this section we give the broad outlines for sound management. But the combination of measures best for you needs to be worked out with your doctor. It has been said that the person who has himself for a doctor has a fool for a patient. In many areas of medicine, and for some kinds of arthritis, this is not true—you can do just as well looking after yourself. But with rheumatoid arthritis you do need a doctor. Indeed, if your rheumatoid arthritis is at all severe, you may want to be seen, at least occasionally, by a specialist in arthritis, a *rheumatologist*.

First, some common sense. Your rheumatoid arthritis may be with you, on and off, for months or years. The best treatments are those that will help you maintain a life that is as nearly normal as possible. Often the worst treatments are those that offer immediate relief. They may allow joint damage to progress or may cause delayed side effects that ultimately make you feel worse. So, you must develop some patience with the disease and with its management. You have to adjust your thinking to operate in the same slow time scale that the disease uses. You and your doctor will want to be anticipating problems before they occur so that they may be avoided. The adjustment to a long-term illness, with the necessity to plan treatment programmes that may take months to get results, is a difficult psychological task. It is easy to understand in principle but hard to put into daily action. This adjustment will be one of your hardest jobs in battling your arthritis.

Synovitis is the underlying problem. The inflammation of the joint membrane releases enzymes that very slowly damage the joint structures. Good treatment reduces this inflammation and stops the damage. Painkillers can increase comfort but do not decrease the arthritis. In fact, pain *per se* helps to protect the joints by discouraging too much use. So, in RA it is important to treat pain by treating the inflammation that causes the pain. By and large, drugs that relieve pain without lessening inflammation must be avoided.

The proper balance between rest and exercise is hard to understand. Rest reduces the inflammation, and this is good. But rest also lets joints get stiff and muscles get weak. With too much rest, tendons become less strong and bones get softer. Obviously, this is bad. So, moderation is the basic principle. It may help you to know that your body usually gives you the right signals about what to do and what not to do. If it hurts too much, don't do it. If you don't seem to have much problem with an activity, go ahead. As a general rule, if you continue to have exercise-caused pain for more than two hours after exercising, you have done too much.

A particularly painful joint may require a splint to help it rest. Still, you will want to exercise the joint by stretching it gently in different directions to keep it from getting stiff. You will not want to use a splint for too long, or you may want to use it just at night. As the joint gets better you will want to begin using the joint, gently at first but slowly progressing to more and more activity. In general, favour activities that build good muscle tone, not those that build great muscle strength. Walking and swimming are better than furniture moving and weight lifting, since tasks requiring a lot of strength put a lot of stress across the joint. And regular exercises done daily are better than occasional sprees of activity that unduly stress joints not ready for so much exertion.

Common sense and a regular, long-term programme are the keys to success. Should you take a nap after lunch? Yes, if you're tired. Should you undertake some particular outing? Go on a trip? You know your regular daily activity level. Common sense will answer most such questions. Full normal activity should be approached gradually with a long-term conditioning programme that includes rest when needed and gradual increases in activity during non-resting periods.

Physiotherapists and occupational therapists can often help with specific advice and helpful hints. The best therapists will help you develop your own programme for home exercise and will teach you the exercises and activities that will help your joints. However, don't expect the therapists to do your programme for you. Your rest and exercise programme cannot consist solely of formal sessions at a rehabilitation facility. You must take the responsibility to build the habits that will, on a daily basis, protect and strengthen your joints. It is important to start exercise and joint protection before you have problems. These are good preventive measures.

Medications are required by most persons with rheumatoid arthritis and often must be continued for months or years. By and large, the most powerful drugs have the worst side effects. So, good physicians will begin with the simplest and the safest drugs and will use more hazardous drugs only if the simpler measures are not sufficient. Most people will not require the more powerful drugs.

Aspirin is the most valuable single drug, when used correctly. Every person with arthritis should know all about aspirin. Aspirin, used correctly, is a strong anti-inflammatory drug with an acceptable level of side effects. Drugs roughly similar to aspirin are called *nonsteroidal anti-inflammatory drugs* and are frequently used. Examples of such drugs are Brufen, Naprosyn and Indocid. (For more information, see Chapter 12.)

Antimalarial drugs such as chloroquine or hydroxychloroquine are sometimes used next, if the anti-inflammatory agents have not been enough. Gold injections are often helpful if the previous drugs have not been sufficient and sometimes result in complete disappearance of the arthritis. Penicillamine is a fairly new drug that also can result in dramatic improvement.

Corticosteroids, most frequently prednisone, are strong hormones with dangerous long-term side effects. Their use is controversial in rheumatoid arthritis; some physicians feel that they should almost never be used, and others use them, but only in very small doses. Immunosuppressant drugs, such as azathioprine (Imuran) and chlorambucil (Leukeran), are powerful, experimental, and hazardous; many physicians think that these drugs are too dangerous to use in rheumatoid arthritis. Steroids and immunosuppressants are sometimes needed for severe complications such as nerve damage or eye damage.

Surgery sometimes can restore the function of a damaged joint. Hip replacement, knee replacement, and synovectomy (removal of the joint membrane) are the most common operations.

3
Osteoarthritis

Osteoarthritis (osteoarthrosis, OA, degenerative joint disease, DJD) is the kind of arthritis that everybody gets. It is a practically universal problem, increasing with age, and one that, because of its relationship to the aging process, is not as responsive to medical treatment as we might like. However, there are many things you can do for yourself to help this disease. Fortunately, osteoarthritis usually is a mild condition. Osteoarthritis is a much less severe form of arthritis than rheumatoid arthritis. In other words, the changes in the skeleton that occur with age are inevitable, but they cause symptoms in a minority of people and severe symptoms in very few.

The tissue involved in osteoarthritis is the cartilage. This is the gristle material that faces the ends of the bones and forms the surface of the joint on both sides. Gristle is tough, somewhat elastic, and very durable. The cartilage or gristle does not have a blood supply, so it gets its oxygen and nutrition from the surrounding joint fluid. In this it is aided by being elastic and by being able to absorb fluid. When we use a joint, the pressure squeezes fluid and waste products out of the cartilage, and when the pressure is relieved, the fluid seeps back, together with oxygen and nutrients. Hence, the health of the cartilage depends on use of the joint. Over many years, the cartilage may become frayed and may even wear away entirely. When this happens, the bone surface on one side of the joint grates against the bone on the other side of the joint, providing a much less elastic joint surface. With time, the opposing bony surfaces may become polished, a process called *eburnation*. As this happens, the joint may again move more smoothly and cause less discomfort. This is one of the reasons it is important to continue to use painful joints.

Osteoarthritis is sometimes called osteoarthrosis. The difference between these two terms has to do with the question of inflammation. *Itis* denotes inflammation, and with osteoarthritis very little inflammation is to be found. Hence, some experts prefer the term osteoarthrosis, which does not imply inflammation. Both words mean the same.

There are three common types of osteoarthritis. The first and mildest causes knobby enlargement of the finger joints. The end joints of the fingers become bony and the hands begin to assume the appearance we associate with old age. The other joints of the fingers may also be involved. This kind of arthritis (or arthrosis) usually causes little difficulty beyond the cosmetic. There may be some stiffness.

The second form of osteoarthritis involves the spine. Bony growths (spurs) appear on the spine in the neck region or in the low back. Usually the bony growths are associated with some narrowing of the space between the vertebrae. This time the disc rather than cartilage is the material that becomes frayed. Changes in the spine begin early in life in almost all of us, but cause symptoms relatively seldom.

The third form of osteoarthritis involves the weight-bearing joints, almost always the hips and knees. These problems can be quite severe. It is possible to have all three kinds of osteoarthritis or any two of them, but often a person will have only one.

Individuals who have had fractures near a joint or have a congenital malformation at a joint seem to develop osteoarthritis in those joints at an earlier age. On the other hand, the usual description of this arthritis as "wear and tear" is not accurate. While excessive wear and tear on the joint can theoretically result in damage, activity helps the joint remain supple and lubricated, and this tends to cancel out the theoretically bad effects.

At any rate, careful studies of people who regularly put a lot of stress on joints (such as individuals who operate pneumatic drills or run long distances on hard paved surfaces) have been unable to show a relationship between these activities and the development of arthritis. Hence, intensive activity does not predispose you to arthritis any more than intensive activity predisposes you to heart disease. In fact, the very opposite may be true.

FEATURES

The bony knobs that form around the end joints of the fingers are called *Heberden's nodes* after the British doctor who first described them. In the middle joints of the fingers, similar knobs can be found. Usually, the bony enlargement occurs slowly over a period of years and is not even noticed. In most cases, all of the fingers are involved more or less equally.

Osteoarthritis of the spine does not cause symptoms unless there is pressure on one of the nerves or irritation of some of the other structures of the back. If someone tells you that you have arthritis in your spine, do not assume that the pain you feel is necessarily related to that arthritis. Most people with X-rays showing arthritis of the spine do not have any problem at all.

Osteoarthritis of the weight-bearing joints, particularly the hip and knee, develops slowly and often involves both sides of the body. Pain in the joint may remain fairly constant or may wax and wane over a period of years. In severe cases walking may be difficult or even impossible. Fluid may accumulate in the affected joint, giving it a swollen appearance, or a knee may wobble a bit when weight is placed on it. Usually, in the knee, the osteoarthritis will affect the inner or the outer half of the joint more than the other; this may result in the leg becoming bowed or splayed and may cause difficulty in walking.

X-rays can be helpful in evaluating osteoarthritis. The two major findings on the X-ray are narrowing of the joint space and the presence of bony spurs. X-rays pass right through cartilage. Hence, in a normal joint the X-ray looks as though the two bones are separated by a space. In reality, the apparent space is filled with cartilage. As the cartilage is frayed, the apparent joint space on the X-ray narrows until the two bones may touch each other. *Osteophytes,* or spurs, are little bone growths that appear alongside the places where the cartilage has degenerated. It is as though the body is trying to react to a cartilage problem by providing more surface area for the joint, so as to distribute the weight more evenly. The bony growth provides a larger joint surface, although the new bone is not covered by cartilage. In addition, X-rays can sometimes show the holes through which the nerves pass and indicate whether these holes are narrowed or not.

In contrast to X-rays, blood tests are not very helpful in diagnosing osteoarthritis. There is not anything wrong with the rest of the body, so all the tests are normal.

PROGNOSIS (THE FUTURE OF THE DISEASE)

Prognosis is good to excellent for all forms of osteoarthritis. When you think of an aging process, you tend to think of a progressive condition that will continue to get worse and worse. That is not necessarily the case. Osteoarthritis may get worse for a while and then become stable for a long time. A joint that has lost its cartilage may not function well at first, but with use the bone may be moulded and polished so that a smooth and more functional joint is developed. Even in the worst cases, osteoarthritis progresses slowly. You have lots of time to think about what kinds of treatment are likely to help. If a surgical decision is needed, you can consider for some time whether you want an operation or not. Crippling from osteoarthritis is relatively rare, and most persons with osteoarthritis remain essentially free of symptoms.

TREATMENT

Joints should be exercised through their full range of motion several times a day. If weight-bearing joints are involved, body weight should be kept under control. Obesity accelerates the rate of damage. The most helpful exercises seem to be swimming, walking, and bicycling, which are easy, can be gradually increased, and are smooth rather than jerky. Exercise should be regular. Thus, if you start getting some osteoarthritis, it is not a signal to begin to tone down your life, but rather to develop a sensible regular exercise program to strengthen the bones and ligaments surrounding the affected joints and to preserve mobility in joints that are developing spurs. (For details see Chapter 5.)

Drug therapy is much less important. We use it to control the discomfort to a certain extent. Aspirin in moderate doses (or paracetamol) is frequently helpful. Indomethacin and other anti-inflammatory drugs may be helpful for some people, particularly if the osteoarthritis is in the hip or the knee. We try to avoid codeine and other strong pain relievers because pain is a signal to the body that helps protect a diseased joint; it is important that this signal is received. (For details see Chapter 12.)

Frequently some kinds of devices can assist. A cane may be helpful; less commonly, crutches are needed. Occasionally, special shoes or lifts on one side of the foot may be helpful.

Most physicians believe that osteoarthritis may be prevented by good health habits. If you are active, maintain a lean body weight, exercise your muscles and joints regularly so as to nourish cartilage, and let your common sense tell you when you have done too much and something hurts, your joints should last a lifetime. Like exercise of the heart muscle, exercise of the muscles and joints provides reserve for the occasional strenuous activities we all encounter. Exercise builds strong tissues that last a long time.

Injection of osteoarthritic joints with corticosteroids is occasionally helpful, and sometimes removal of some fluid from a joint may help. Unfortunately, injections usually do not help much since there is not much inflammation to be suppressed. Injections should not be frequently repeated, because the injection itself may damage the cartilage and the bone.

Surgery can be dramatically effective for persons with severe osteo-arthritis of the weight-bearing joints. The total hip replacement operation is the most important operation yet devised for any form of arthritis. Practically all individuals are free of pain after the surgery and many walk normally and carry out normal activities. The total knee replacement is a more recent operation that already gives far better results than the knee surgery available just a few years ago. Surgery is not required on an urgent basis, and you and your doctor will want to decide the point at which the discomfort or the limitation of your walking has become sufficiently great so that the discomfort and the small risk associated with the operation are warranted.

4
Those Nagging Pains
BURSITIS AND GETTING OLD

Most of the problems we tend to call arthritis don't even involve the joint and really aren't even diseases. This is good news. Painful local conditions involving only one or two parts of the body are almost always just an irritation or injury of that part. After that part is rested or fixed everything is all right again. There is no crippling, no threat to life, no need for dangerous medications. Remember the basic principle: For a local problem use a local treatment. Very seldom will you want to take a medication by mouth for a pain in, say, an elbow.

There are a lot of names for these conditions—bursitis, low back strain, sciatica, metatarsalgia, Achilles tendinitis, heel-spur syndrome, sprained ankle, cervical neck strain, frozen shoulder, tennis elbow, housemaid's knee, carpal-tunnel syndrome, and others. Many people call all of these bursitis, while doctors have other and fancier names for them. But they all are local conditions and are first approached the same way. At first you don't even need a doctor for them, but if they don't respond after six weeks of self-treatment or seem alarmingly severe, be sure to see the doctor.

BURSITIS

A bursa is a small sac of tissue similar to the synovial tissue that lines the joints. The bursa sac contains a lubricating fluid, and the bursa is designed to ease the movement of muscle across muscle or of muscle across bone. A bursa does not connect to the joint space of the nearby joint but is a separate sac. In the grand scheme of things the bursa is just an annoying little body area, but bursae can be very painful when they become inflamed. Usually, only one or two will be inflamed at a time, but bursitis of over 20 bursae can occur, and the problems can come and go over the years.

"Housemaid's knee" is a popular term for *prepatellar bursitis*, in which the bursa in front and just below the kneecap is inflamed. *Olecranon bursitis* occurs over the point of the elbow, and sometimes a fluid-filled sac is visible at that point. *Subdeltoid bursitis* occurs at the shoulder, or more precisely, on the outer aspect of the upper arm just below the shoulder.

Features

Bursitis is inflammation of a bursa and results in localized pain. Sometimes the pain is on both sides of the body, as with both knees. There is pain when the inflamed area is pressed, and heat and redness are common. If the bursa is located close enough to the skin, swelling can be seen. Many bursae, however, are buried deep between muscles.

Bursitis comes on relatively suddenly, within hours to days. It frequently follows injury to the area, repeated pressure on the area, or overuse. In the shoulders, particularly, it may be associated with inflammation of the tendon and can be part of a "frozen shoulder" problem.

Prognosis

Almost all episodes of bursitis will subside within several days to several weeks, but may recur. If the process causing the bursitis is continued, the bursitis may persist, otherwise it follows a normal healing course over a period of one week to ten days. Some people seem more prone to bursitis than others and have recurrent problems throughout their lives. If the affected part is held rigid, some permanent stiffness may result; otherwise no crippling whatsoever should result from bursitis.

Treatment

If the problem is tolerable, treat it with "tincture of time." Wait for the body to control and heal the process. Avoid the precipitating cause. Use drugs very sparingly; the process is local and systemic drugs like aspirin are not very helpful. Resting the part will speed the healing, and you may want to use a sling or other device to increase the rest. Gentle warmth provided by a heating pad or warm bath frequently makes the bursitis feel better. The affected area should be worked through its full range of motion two to four times a day, even if it is a bit tender, to prevent stiffness from developing. Additional techniques described in Chapter 8 may also be helpful. But remember, patience and avoidance of reinjury are the major tactics.

If the discomfort persists for a number of weeks despite the measures outlined above, see the doctor. Often, the doctor will recommend that you continue the same general measures discussed here. Alternatively, an anti-inflammatory drug may be prescribed; these help few people and are generally just a way of buying a little more patience from the patient. Finally, the doctor may inject the bursa with corticosteroids (see Chapter 12). These injections are usually successful and not overly painful. They are relatively free of side effects and most physicians feel that they are appropriate treatment for a local condition that is severe and persistent.

GETTING OLD

Local injuries, like bursitis, are often dismissed as "just getting old, I suppose." It is true that more older people than younger people have these problems, and they do have something to do with the way that our bodies age.

But they do not need to happen. These problems are sometimes due to abuse of a body part, as in prepatellar bursitis from scrubbing floors on your knees. Much more frequently, however, they are due to disuse. In our society, as you get older you are expected to be less active. And then you get the kinds of health problems that happen to inactive people of all ages. The relationship between local problems and age is mostly accidental; it is really an association of local problems with inactivity.

So you need to be active. If your muscles are trim and in good tone, your heart and lungs are conditioned, your body weight is normal and constant at that level, and you have a regular exercise programme you will have far fewer of these problems, and your body will not grow old as rapidly. These measures will keep calcium in your bones, your bursae free and well lubricated, your tendons firm and strong, and your joint cartilage well nourished.

You can control a lot of the aging of your body. The worst mistake that you can make is to consider bursitis or another local problem to be a signal to slow down. It is a signal to speed up, because your body is drifting out of condition. In the next chapter we go through some of the exercises that will help.

5

Use It or Lose It
EXERCISES FOR YOUR ARTHRITIS

One of the most important things you can do to help your arthritis is to exercise, if you do it right. Unfortunately, many people with arthritis think exercise is harmful. Others become discouraged because progress is slow or their exercises are painful. Maintaining a proper balance between rest and exercise and exercising properly are the keys to a successful arthritis exercise programme. Let us examine the benefits of exercise, some basic principles, and the different types of exercise. With this knowledge you can plan a successful and enjoyable programme.

BENEFITS OF EXERCISE

There are numerous benefits of exercise, touching many aspects of our physical and psychological lives. It is well known that exercise leads to increased strength and flexibility in the muscles and ligaments surrounding the joints. In addition, research has shown that exercise helps to maintain or increase the strength of bone. More dynamic forms of exercise, such as swimming or walking, have important effects on the heart that promote increased endurance and circulation and fight deterioration of the arteries.

Every tissue in the body requires certain foods or nutrients to work effectively. Most tissues have arteries that bring essential foods to them, but this is not true of the joint cartilage. It is only through movement that nourishment is brought by the synovial fluid to the joint cartilage and that waste products are removed. Thus, exercise promotes good joint nutrition.

An appropriate exercise programme can lead to a general sense of well-being and accomplishment. It is easy to feel good about yourself when you are accomplishing the goals of a realistic exercise programme. Further, the social interactions encouraged by many forms of exercise are also rewarding.

Exercise is a way we can prevent the loss of function that may accompany arthritis. There is a saying that applies particularly to persons with arthritis: "Use it or lose it." If you do not use a muscle or joint you will lose strength and mobility, and thus, function. If loss of function has already occurred, it is important to remember that it was not lost in one day. Likewise, it cannot be regained in one day. Slow progress is to be expected, particularly if your arthritis is severe or your joint limitations have existed for a long time. Expect some setbacks in any exercise programme but keep at it. Your efforts will be rewarded in many ways.

PRINCIPLES OF EXERCISE

When Should I Exercise?

Exercises should be done daily for the rest of your life. It is the "weekend warrior" who gets into trouble with painful strained muscles and ligaments. The only time a joint should not be exercised is when it is inflamed, or "hot" (swollen, red, tender to the touch). The "hot" joint is one of the special exercise considerations for people with rheumatoid arthritis. However, even those hot joints should be gently moved through the full range of motion twice a day.

Find a specific time and place to exercise and make this a part of your daily routine. You will have to decide on the best time, but consider the following: It is best to exercise when (1) you have the least pain, (2) you have the least stiffness, (3) you are not tired, and (4) your medication is having maximum effect. You probably want one such period early in the day, and one later.

What Can I Do to Prepare for Exercise?

Athletes learn that warming up before exercise means a more productive session and helps prevent injuries. Here are some warm-up suggestions.

1. A nice, slow general stretch: Lying in bed, (a) stretch one arm up and then the other, (b) push arms forward, opening hands wide, (c) pull arms

back and close hands, (d) pull knees up and do a few bicycle turns in the air, (e) stretch legs out straight, (f) roll to the side, swinging legs off the edge of the bed, using momentum to help you sit up. This warm-up is helpful when first getting up in the morning and is very similar to what a cat does as it gets up from a rest.

2. Begin your exercise programme with small movements in a pain-free range. These movements can be anything from your chosen exercise done less vigorously to a good shake (like a dog shaking). Before walking or jogging do some gentle stretching of the leg muscles.

3. Massage can be used to relax stiff joints and muscles prior to exercise. However, it is best not to deeply massage a "hot" joint.

4. Apply heat prior to exercise. Heat tends to relax joints and muscles and relieve pain. How you apply the heat is up to you. No way is better than another. You do not need special equipment or mineral waters. All of the following are acceptable ways of applying heat. When using heat always test carefully for temperature (the elbow is a good tester) to avoid burns.

   a) Take a long, hot bath. A hot spring, whirlpool bath, or hot tub is nice, but not necessary. Use caution and stand up slowly as the heat sometimes causes dizziness.

   b) Take a long, hot shower and aim the full force of the water at the painful joint(s). Hand-held showers with a massage unit can be pleasant.

   c) An electric heating pad can be placed over the affected area. Be sure the hot pad has a cover and that you do not fall asleep with it plugged in. It is best not to lie directly on the pad, and never use an electric pad with anything wet.

   d) Fill a hot-water bottle with hot water. Be sure it is not hot enough to burn you. Again, it is best not to lie directly on the water bottle.

   e) Stand next to your heater or radiator.

5. If you don't get good results from heat, the application of cold may prove more effective, especially for the "hot" joint of rheumatoid arthritis. Cold relaxes muscles and produces a numbing effect, thus decreasing pain and increasing joint motion. As with heat, there are a few important principles of application:

   a) If you are especially sensitive to cold or have decreased sensation or circulation such as in Raynaud's Disease or vasculitis, do not apply cold. Ask your doctor or therapist if you are unsure.

   b) Apply just long enough to achieve a numbing effect—no more than 15 to 20 minutes.

c) Be cautious when exercising after applying cold; the numbing effect may allow you to overdo it. Remember, if the joint is "hot," restrict exercise to moving the joint through its full range of motion twice a day.

d) Place the cold pack over the joint, not between the joint and a firm surface.

e) Check during and after application for any sign of a break in the skin.

Cold packs can be bought, or you can create your own. Wrapping the pack in a warm, moist towel will help you adjust to the cold. Use whichever cold pack method is easiest and most effective for you:

a) Several resourceful people have suggested a sack of frozen peas! You can refreeze it and use it again.

b) Massage with a large ice cube.

c) Make a slush pack: Line a bowl with two heavy plastic bags; fill with three cups water and one cup denatured alcohol. Fasten the bags and place the bowl in the freezer until slush forms. You can refreeze a slush pack.

How Should I Exercise?

Be consistent and stick to your chosen set of exercises. Begin at a comfortable level for you and gradually increase the number of repetitions. Progress more slowly with rheumatoid joints that are prone to "hot" periods. With this gradual progression you will avoid unnecessary pain.

Your exercises should minimize stress on the affected joints. Carefully assess the stress each exercise imposes on the priority joint and those surrounding it. You will find further discussion of this throughout the chapter.

Exercises for arthritis should be performed with a slow, steady rhythm. Give your muscles time to relax between repetitions of each exercise (10 to 15 seconds). After a muscle is used, it must relax and lengthen so that waste products of muscle action can be carried away. Learning to relax readily and completely during exercise will make any exercise programme more effective and enjoyable. Techniques aimed at release of residual tension throughout the body will be discussed in Chapter 8.

It is important to coordinate your breathing with exercise. Breathe deeply and rhythmically as you exercise; never hold your breath. Interspersing deep breathing with exercise ensures an adequate oxygen supply to working muscles as well as release of tension. Deep breathing involves inhaling slowly and gently through your nose and drawing air down into your abdomen. Hold for at least five counts. Exhale slowly and gently through lightly closed lips for at least five counts. You can do this breathing exercise in between the exercises described later.

What Should I Avoid?

Remember that your exercises should minimize stress on the joints. Avoid high-tension exercises such as weight lifting. If your weight-bearing joints are affected (hips, knees, ankles, or spine), jogging should be approached cautiously. Bicycling for a painful knee should also be approached with caution: set a stationary bicycle on the lowest resistance or use a low gear on a conventional bicycle.

If a chosen exercise for one joint places excessive stress on another involved joint—for example, a shoulder exercise that stresses an involved hand, or a hip exercise that stresses a painful low back—modify the exercise or substitute another.

As stated earlier, avoid exercising the hot, inflamed joint, but remember to move it through its full range of motion twice a day. Deep massage of the painful joint should also be avoided. Never take extra medication to mask joint pain before exercising. This could result in joint damage, as pain is your real guide to when you've done too much.

Since warmth helps relax stiff muscles and joints, avoid becoming chilled during exercise. Wear warm clothing and do not exercise in a draft or a cold room. Hand exercises can be done in a basin of warm water.

When Have I Done Too Much?

Use common sense and listen to the signals your body gives you. A general rule of thumb is that if exercise-induced pain lasts longer than two hours, cut back. Do not stop. The key here is "exercise-induced." If you do your exercises and then go out and garden for three hours the chances are that the prolonged gardening is responsible for any residual pain.

Any exercise programme is bound to have setbacks, but these are not permanent. If you experience exercise-induced pain for longer than two hours, decrease the number of repetitions or be less forceful. If that does not help, choose a different exercise that will achieve the same result but that is more appropriate for you. Also, review the principles of exercise discussed here and in the sections on stretching and strengthening exercises.

TYPES OF EXERCISE

There are three basic types of exercise. **Range-of-motion** or **stretching exercises** involve moving a joint as far as it will comfortably go (through its full range of motion) and then coaxing it a little farther, just past the point of beginning pain or discomfort. These exercises are designed to increase and then maintain joint mobility, thus decreasing pain and improving function.

Strengthening exercises increase muscle strength and thus lend stability to vulnerable joints. They improve your ability to bear weight, lift objects, and sustain movement. Strengthening exercises should be done in such a way as to minimize stress on the joints. For this reason, good strengthening exercises are *isometric*. These exercises involve use (contraction) of a muscle or muscles without movement at the joint. Discussion and examples of the isometric principle can be found in the section on specific strengthening exercises. Remember, strengthening exercises are not a substitute for stretching exercises. They will not increase joint range of motion.

Endurance exercises are necessary because neither stretching nor strengthening exercises will increase your endurance. More dynamic forms of exercise, such as walking, swimming, bicycling, jogging, dancing, or cross-country skiing will promote cardiovascular fitness. Include some kind of dynamic exercise in your programme every day, but remember to start out easy and progress slowly. To help reduce stress while walking or dancing wear low-heeled, rubber-soled, lightweight shoes. A good running shoe is essential for any runner with joint or muscle problems; try them on before you buy and consult a running guide for current recommendations. These are often excellent shoes for just walking.

STRETCHING OR RANGE-OF-MOTION EXERCISES

The general rule for stretching exercises is to move the joint as far as it will comfortably go (its full range of motion) and then coax it a little further, just past the point of first pain. Do not "bounce." A gentle, sustained stretch will be less stressful to your joints and more effective. **Each stretching exercise should be repeated three to ten times, two to four times a day, depending on pain.** Remember one of the basic principles of exercise as you decide on the number of repetitions—start slow and easy. If you have exercise-induced pain lasting longer than two hours, cut back a little. Don't give up.

The exercises in this section are examples of stretching exercises. As you become familiar with the principles involved, you may want to design your own exercises or incorporate others you have learned.

Before proceeding to the exercises, take a mental survey of your joints. To maintain your present function, you must move every joint in your body through its full range of motion every day. This movement usually occurs during your daily activities. However, because of your arthritis you may be protecting some joints by not moving them. Do you have joints that are not moved through their full range of motion every day or joints that you cannot move as far as you used to? If so, please list them here.

1.

2.

3.

4.

5.

It is difficult to stretch more than two or three joints at a time. Choose two or three priority joints with which to start working and pick a goal for each joint. For example:

1. **Shoulder.** I want to reach above my head to touch the top shelf.
2. **Fingers.** I want to touch the tips of my fingers to my palm.

MY PRIORITY JOINTS   *MY GOAL*

1.

2.

3.

Once you have reached your goal for one of these joints, you can then add stretching exercises for another. But remember, to maintain the mobility that you worked so hard to achieve you must move that joint through its full range of motion once or twice a day. If you notice that you are losing ground with that joint, then resume a more concentrated stretching programme.

Now, turn to the appropriate stretching exercises for your priority joints.

HANDS

The hand is a very delicate and intricate part of the body. The following exercises will help maintain or increase movements essential to the skilled movements we perform with our hands. If you have severe hand deformity or involvement you may wish to consult an occupational therapist or physiotherapist in developing your initial programme. Also, when choosing exercises for other parts of the body, remember to assess the stress imposed on the hands and modify the exercise if necessary. See Chapter 6 for suggestions on how to modify activities to protect the involved hand.

1. One-Two-Three Finger Exercise

For optimum function you should be able to touch the tips of your fingers to the palm. When stretching the fingertips toward the palm use the "one-two-three" approach. Begin with the joint closest to the tip of the finger (A), then move on to the middle joint (B). When your fingertips are touching the palm or as close as possible, bend the knuckle joint (C). You may exercise your fingers individually or together, using your other hand to guide the movement if necessary.

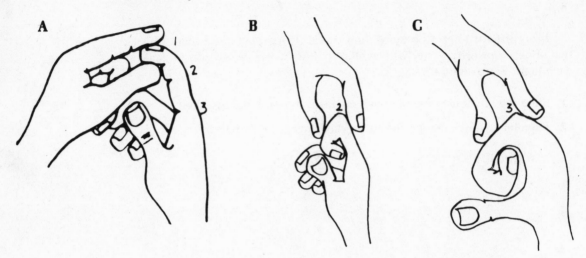

2. Three-Two-One Finger Exercise

If any of the joints in your fingers will not straighten completely, try this exercise, which is the reverse of 1. With you fingertips as close to the palm as possible, begin to uncurl your hand. Begin with the knuckle joint (A), move to the middle joint (B), and finally exercise the joint closest to the tip of the finger (C).

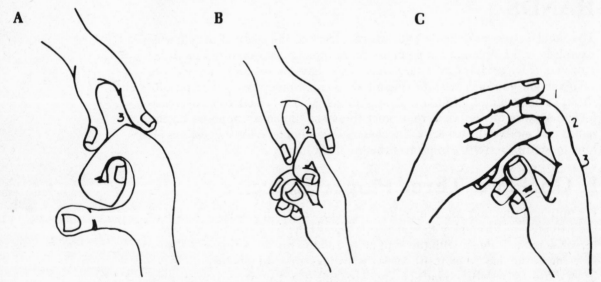

3. Fingers Flat Exercise

This is another exercise for straightening the joints of the fingers. Lay your hand as flat as possible on a table. Place the heel of your other hand across your fingers and gently press down, straightening the fingers.

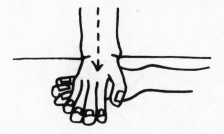

4. The Thumb Walk

Try to form a letter "O" with each attempt of this exercise. Lightly touch the tip of the thumb to the tip of the index finger (A), then spread your fingers as wide as you can (B). Proceed on to touch the tip of the thumb to the tips of your other fingers, spreading the fingers wide after each attempt. If you cannot quite bring the thumb to touch the finger, use the other hand to coax them closer together.

A

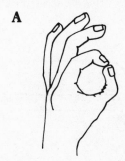

B

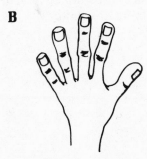

WRISTS

The next two exercises will help maintain or improve your ability to move the wrist back and forth.

5. The Palm Press

First, place your hands together, palms touching and fingers straight (A). Press the right hand backward with the left hand (B), then reverse and press the left hand backward with the right hand. Exert pressure at the palm, *not* the fingertips. Coax the hand just past the point of discomfort.

A   B

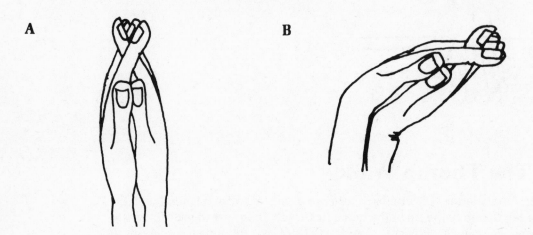

6. Wrist Table Stretch

For a more vigorous wrist stretch hang the hand over the edge of a table or arm rest with the palm down. Raise the hand up as far as possible, using your other hand to assist with the stretch (A). Then lower the hand, stretching just past the point of discomfort (B).

A   B

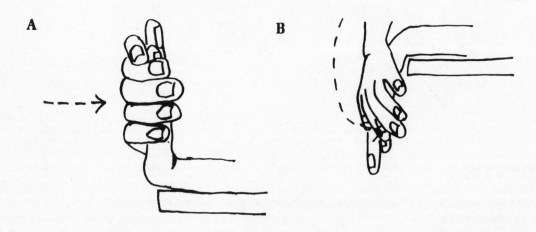

7. The Slide

If you notice that your fingers drift toward the little finger side of the hand (a common deformity in rheumatoid arthritis), this exercise is for you. Place your forearm on a table, palm down. Slide each finger toward the thumb, not moving the forearm. Use your other hand to assist if necessary. Repeat with the other hand. The exercise works to keep your knuckles and wrist in correct alignment with your forearm, promoting optimum function.

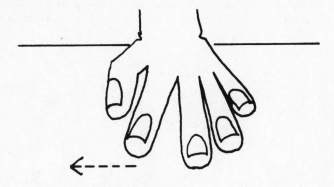

8. The Door Opener

This is an exercise to stretch the muscles and ligaments that rotate the forearm, allowing you to turn doorknobs and unlock doors. Start with your forearm resting on a table, palm down. Turn your hand so the palm faces up (A). If you use your other hand to assist with the stretch, grasp the lower part of the forearm, not the hand.

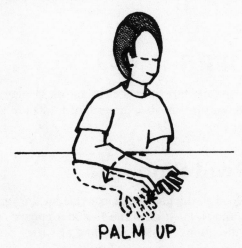

PALM UP

ELBOWS

9. The Elbow Chop

The diagonal pattern in this exercise is similar to that of chopping wood and is designed to help you bend and straighten the elbow completely. Place hands together and bend both elbows until your hands touch your right shoulder (A). Then bring hands down to touch the left knee, straightening elbows completely (B). Remember to coax the elbow a little farther than it wants to go. Reverse directions, going from left shoulder to right knee.

A

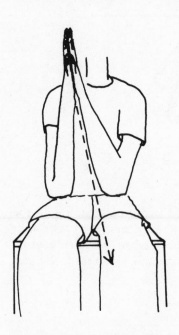

B

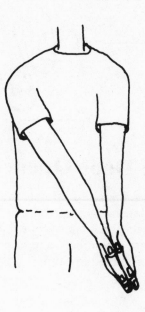

SHOULDERS

The shoulder is one of those joints that moves in many directions. When choosing stretching exercises, it is important to decide which functions are most important to you.

10. The Pendulum

This exercise is good as the beginning exercise for the very painful or limited shoulder. It facilitates relaxation of the shoulder muscles as well as free joint movement in all directions. From a standing or sitting position, lean slightly forward. Let your arm hang freely in front of you. Relax and feel the weight of your arm. Keeping the arm straight, begin with small circles and gradually increase their size. Remember to exercise to just past the point of discomfort. Don't get carried away with your circles.

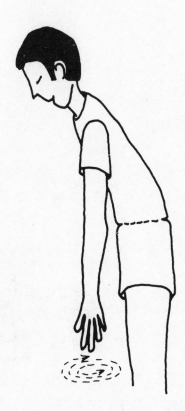

11. The Shoulder Rotator

If you have difficulty touching the back of your neck, combing your hair, or zipping a back zipper, then you probably need to work on outward rotation of the shoulder. Here are two ways to accomplish this movement. (A) Clasp your hands together at the back of your neck and pull the elbows as far back as possible. You should feel a stretch at the front of the shoulder and chest. (B) If you are not yet ready for the first exercise, begin with this method.

Hold your arm close to your side with elbow bent. Keeping elbow at your side, rotate hand and forearm outward as far away from your stomach as possible. You may use your other hand to assist with the stretch.

A

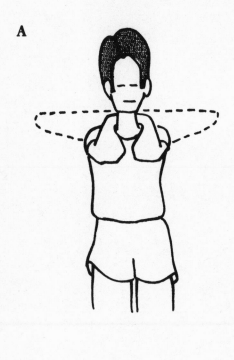

B

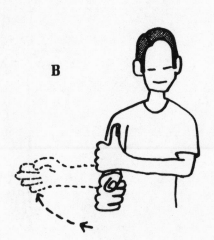

Here are three exercises to increase your ability to reach overhead. This is important for dressing, getting things off shelves, or picking apples. You do not need to do all of these exercises. One exercise repeated three to ten times, two to four times a day, is sufficient. Pick the one that suits you best, or change exercises occasionally for variety.

12. The Shoulder Cradle

If your shoulder is still very painful, this exercise may be better tolerated. With your arm supported at the elbow by the opposite hand (A), raise the arm up over your head. You can rest your forearm on your head as you coax your shoulder just past the point of pain (B). This exercise may be easier lying down.

A

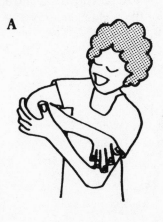

B

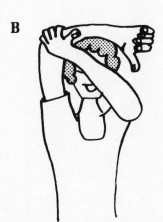

13. The Wand Exercise

Use a cane, yardstick, or mop handle as your wand. Place one hand on each end and raise the wand as high overhead as possible. You might try doing this in front of a mirror. You don't have to move both ends to the same height —play around with it. If holding the wand causes pain in your hand, try building up the grip area as described in Chapter 6 (Principle 8b).

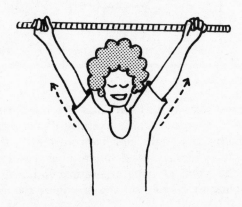

14. The Shoulder Pulley

Throw a piece of rope over the top of an open door, creating a modified pulley system. Hold one end of the rope in each hand. As you pull down on one end, the other arm will be raised up. Coax the arm a little higher than it wants to go and then pull down, raising the opposite arm.

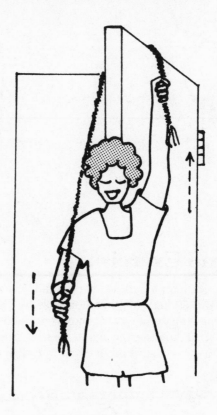

HIPS

The hip is the largest joint of the body and like the shoulder can move in several directions. In choosing which exercise to do, decide which movements are most limited or painful and concentrate on them initially. You should do the selected exercises three to ten times, two to four times a day. Stretch just past the point of pain. If exercise-induced pain persists for longer than two hours after exercise, you are doing too much. *Do not stop, just cut back.*

15. The Spread Eagle

This exercise increases hip motion to the side, which is necessary for riding a bicycle, getting in and out of a car, or riding a horse. Lie on your back. Spread your legs as far apart as possible and then coax them a little farther. You might want someone to measure the distance between your knees so you can keep track of your progress. If this is difficult or if you feel discomfort in your lower back, move one leg at a time while keeping the other leg bent.

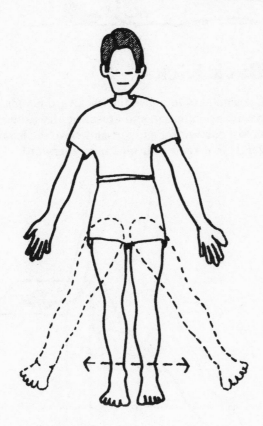

16. Knee-to-Chest

This exercise will help increase the hip motion forward, which is important for activities such as walking, climbing stairs, and getting on and off low furniture. Lie on your back. Keep one leg straight and bring your other knee toward your chest. You can place your hands under the thigh to assist with the stretch. This exercise also helps to stretch the low back. You may want to begin with your other leg slightly bent to decrease strain on the low back.

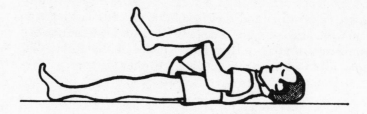

17. The Back Kick

This exercise is designed to increase the backward motion of the hip, which is important for walking, running, and cross-country skiing. From a standing position, hold on to a counter for support and move the leg up and back, knee straight. Start gently and keep your hips facing forward.

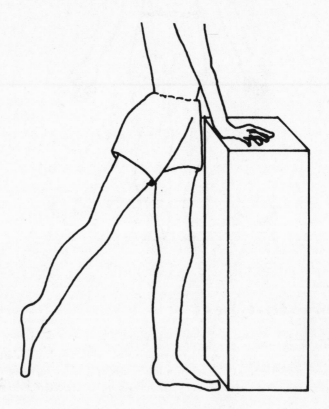

18. The Leg Lift

If you cannot stand up to do the Back Kick, this exercise also helps to increase the backward motion of the hip. Lie face down. This alone may provide a good stretch for those who spend a great deal of time sitting or in bed. If this position is comfortable, raise your leg as high as possible. This exercise should not be done by people with low back or disc problems.

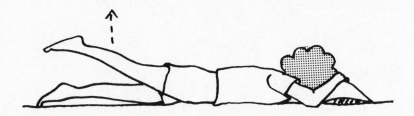

19. The Hip Rotator

This exercise increases the ability of the hip to rotate (roll in and out). This is important for activities such as dancing or rolling over and getting out of bed. Lie on your back, hands out to the side or behind your head. Bend your hips and knees and place feet flat. Cross your right leg over the left knee (A). Rotate hips to the right, trying to touch the knee to the floor (B). Keep your upper body flat on the floor. Repeat to the other side. This is also a good exercise for stretching the low and middle back, but some may find it too strenuous for the back.

A

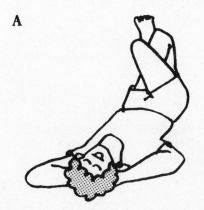

B

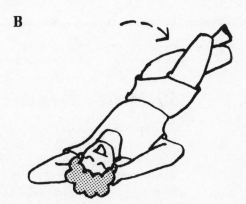

KNEES

The knee is subject to a lot of stress due to its weight-bearing duties and limited muscular support. When stretching the knee it is important to minimize the stress on the joint. Thus you should not be standing when you exercise your knees as the weight of your body adds stress.

The next two exercises are designed to increase your ability to bend and straighten the knee, which is important for climbing stairs or getting up and down from a chair, and most important for standing and walking without fatigue.

20. Knee Bend 1

Lie on your back with both knees bent, feet flat. Bring your knee toward your chest. Using your hands to assist, gently bend the knee, trying to touch your heel to your buttock.

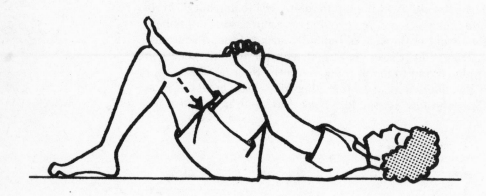

21. Knee Bend 2

If exercise 20 doesn't suit you, try this one. Sit on a straight-backed chair and bend your knee as far back as possible. (Be sure that it is not a part of the chair that keeps you from going farther). To get an extra stretch, place your hands on the side of the chair and shuffle forward toward the edge, keeping your feet in the same position.

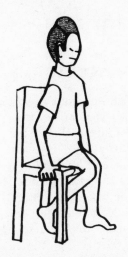

22. The Knee Straightener

The ability to straighten the knee is very important for walking or any standing activity. When one spends a lot of time sitting, the muscles and ligaments in the back of the knee tend to tighten, making it difficult to completely straighten the knee. This exercise is designed to stretch these tissues with a minimum of stress on the joints. Sitting in a straight-backed chair, place your foot on a chair or high footstool. Bend the knee slightly and then straighten by pushing the back of the knee toward the floor. If you find this easy, add another stretch. Place the support. Carefully lean forward; keep your back straight. You will feel a stretch along the hamstring muscles on the back of your leg.

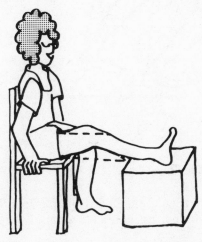

ANKLES AND FEET

23. The Achilles Stretch

This exercise is designed to stretch your Achilles tendon, which is the large tendon you feel at the back of your ankle. It is important to maintain flexibility in this tendon for standing and walking. Joggers should be sure to stretch this tendon before starting out.

Stand at the end of a table and hold onto the sides. Bend the knee of the leg you are not stretching so it almost touches the table. Put the leg to be stretched behind you, keeping both feet flat on the floor. Now lean forward, keeping your back knee straight. You should feel a good stretch in the calf of the leg. This exercise can also be done leaning against a wall or fence.

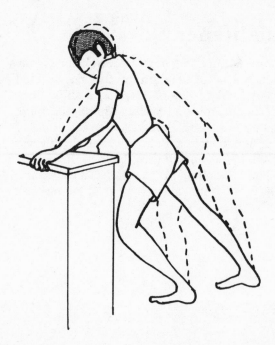

24. The Heel-Toe

Sit in a chair or on the edge of the bed with both feet flat on the floor. First, raise your toes and forefeet as high as you can, keeping your heels on the floor (A). Then, keep your toes on the floor and raise your heels as high as you can (B). This stretches tendons, calf muscles, and the ankle joints.

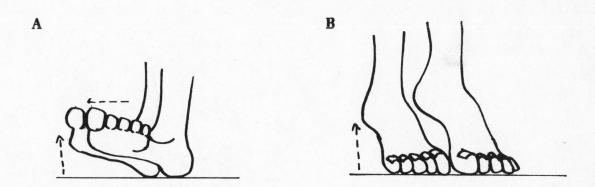

25. The Heel-Toe Dance

Sit in a chair with your feet flat on the ground. With heels on the floor, lift feet and toes as high as you can (A). Keeping the heels on the floor, move feet and toes to the right (B). Then come up on your toes as high as you can and move your heels to the right (C). Reverse and walk feet to the left in the same manner. This helps the rotation at the ankle.

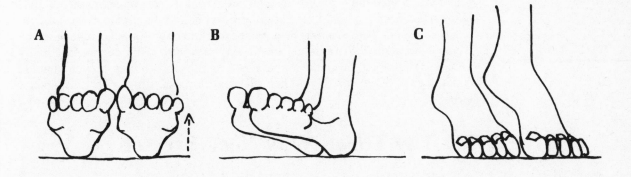

26. The Foot Roll

Place a dowel (large mop handle, closet rod, rolling pin) under the arch of the foot and roll it back and forth. This feels great and it stretches the ligaments of the arch of the foot.

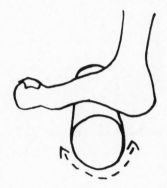

NECK

The neck involves many joints that work together to allow movement. It is one of the easiest parts of the body to exercise. However, it is important to be gentle when you exercise the neck. If you have learned to do neck exercises using circular motions, be sure you only make a half-circle in each direction. A complete circle may cause severe pain for people with bone spurs or a disc problem. If you have found circular exercises to be unsatisfactory, the following exercises should be more appropriate, and we prefer them.

If your neck pain is a new occurrence and the pain is moderate to severe, if you have pain that radiates down your arm with neck movement, or if numbness, tingling, or marked weakness are present in the arm, you should consult your doctor or physiotherapist before proceeding with these exercises.

27. The Three-Way Neck Stretch

1. Relax and slowly drop your chin to your chest, then slowly raise your head and very gently drop the head backward. Do not proceed with this

exercise if you feel a sharp pain or pain down your arm. Return head to the upright position slowly. This motion should never be forced.

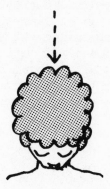
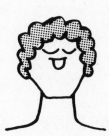

2. Turn to look over your right shoulder, then turn to look as far over the left shoulder as possible.

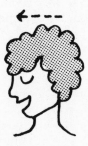
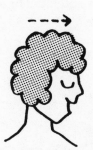

3. Tilt your head to the right and then to the left. Try to touch your ear to your shoulder.

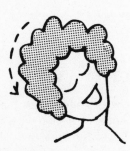
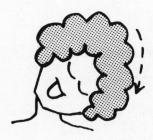

BACK

The following are a series of exercises for those with chronic back problems, especially those with ankylosing spondylitis or generalized stiffness. If your back pain is a new occurrence and the pain is moderate to severe, you should consult your doctor or physiotherapist before proceeding with these exercises. Also, if you notice pain that radiates down your leg, numbness, tingling, or marked weakness, consult a doctor. If exercise-induced pain lasts longer than two hours, cut back a little. Those with ankylosing spondylitis will want to do deep-breathing exercises in addition to ensure good mobility of the rib cage.

28. The Pelvic Tilt

This exercise should be the beginning point for the person with low back problems. Lie on the bed or floor with both knees bent, feet flat. Place your hands on your abdomen. Flatten the small of your back against the floor by tightening your buttocks and pulling in your stomach. If this concept is difficult for you, think of bringing your pubic bone toward your chin. Once you have mastered the pelvic tilt in the lying position, try it while standing and sitting.

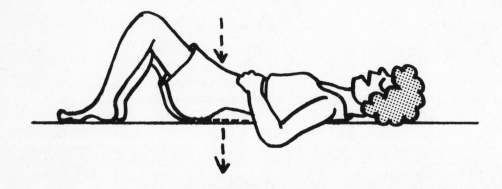

29. Knee-to-Chin Stretch

For a nice low back stretch, lie on the floor with knees bent, feet flat. Bring one knee toward your chin, using your hands to assist with the stretch. Maintain this position for five seconds and lower the leg slowly. Repeat with the other knee. To stretch the upper and middle back at the same time, raise your head and shoulder from the floor as you bring your knee toward your chin. If this creates or increases neck pain, discontinue this portion of the exercise.

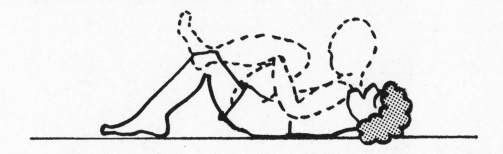

30. The Low Back Rock

Lie on your back with your knees bent and feet flat. Pull knees up to chest, one at a time, grasping under the thighs to assist with the stretch. Rest in this position for five seconds, then gently rock knees from one side to the other, keeping upper back and shoulders on the floor.

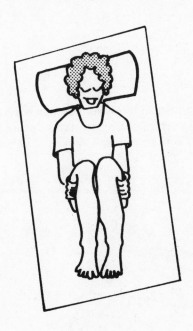
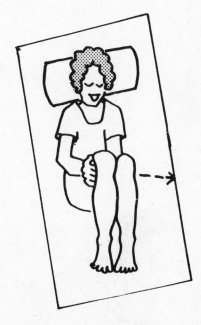

31. The Shoulder-Blade Pinch

This is a good exercise for the middle and upper back. Sit on the edge of a bed or chair. Pinch your shoulder blades together by moving your elbows as far back as possible.

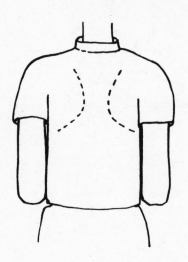
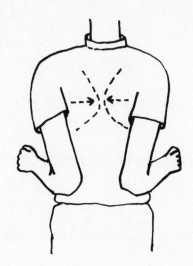

32. The Back Lift

Another way to improve flexibility of the spine is to lie on your stomach. Raise up onto your forearms. If you feel no discomfort, raise up onto extended arms. This exercise should be avoided by people with moderate to severe low back pain.

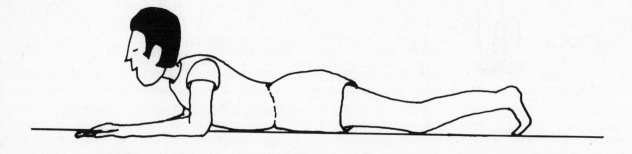

33. The Cat

This exercise should not be done by persons with severe knee, ankle, or hand problems because it places stress on these joints. Assume a crawling position on all fours, with knees bent, arms straight. Taking a deep breath, arch your back as a frightened cat does. Then slowly drop the arch, exhaling completely.

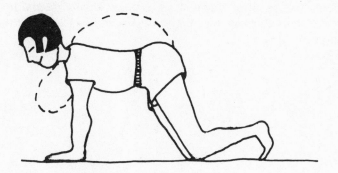

STRENGTHENING EXERCISES

The purpose of these exercises is to maintain strong muscles and to strengthen muscles with as little stress on the joints as possible. Many of them are examples of isometric exercise. If you understand the principles of isometric exercise, you can devise your own exercise for any muscle group. These exercises will not maintain or increase joint mobility.

As described earlier, isometric exercise involves use (contraction) of a muscle with no movement of the joint. One way to accomplish this is to use the muscle to pull or push against a stationary object. The stationary object may be anything from a wall to a body part to an exercise belt. For example, place your hand on the wall and push. You can feel the muscles in your arm working; however, no movement of the joints is taking place. This is an isometric exercise. Here's another example: Sit in a chair and place your right hand on your right knee. Press your right knee against the hand, allowing no movement of the arm or leg. You have used another body part as the stationary object.

One nice thing about isometric exercises is that you do not have to do many to receive the benefits. Each exercise, held for a count of six seconds, three to four times a day, is sufficient. *Gradually* tense and relax the muscle, avoiding sudden, quick movement. To prevent the tendency to hold your breath, count the six seconds out loud. If exercise-induced pain lasts longer than two hours, cut back a little. As with the famous tortoise, slow and steady wins the race. Long, sustained isometric exercise is not advisable for heart patients, but the following exercises should not be harmful. If in doubt, consult your doctor.

For these exercises you will need an exercise belt of some kind. It is best if this belt has some give to it. The inner tube from a bicycle tyre, a shock cord (holds packages on bicycles), or a strong stretch belt will do fine. If all else fails, an ordinary leather belt will suffice. The exercise belt is a closed loop, 30 to 48 inches in circumference.

Before proceeding to specific exercises, take a mental inventory of your body. Are there parts of your body you would like to strengthen? If so, define which parts.

1.

2.

3.

4.

5.

Now pick two or three priorities and proceed to the section dealing with your priority areas. Remember, your goal is not to do every strengthening exercise in the book but to use the ones you specifically need.

1.

2.

3.

HANDS

34. The Finger Press

To strengthen the muscles that bend the fingers and help you pick up objects, try this exercise. Lightly press the tip of the thumb to the tip of the index finger. Hold for six seconds, maintaining a perfect "O" shape, then relax. Continue, lightly pressing the tip of the thumb to the tip of each finger. To help maintain the "O" shape, place a pill bottle or other cylinder in your hand. Those with rheumatoid arthritis should not press the fingers together but just touch them lightly.

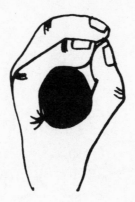

35. The Finger Lift

To strengthen the muscles that straighten the fingers, lay your hand flat on a table. Lay your other hand across the fingers to be exercised. Lift the fingers of the bottom hand, pushing against the top hand. Hold for six seconds; relax. If you have significant weakness, do each finger separately. You should exert only gentle pressure for this exercise.

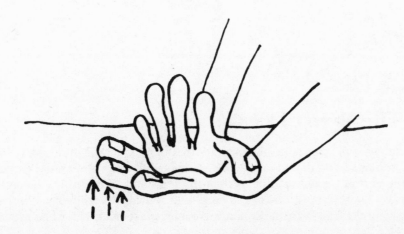

36. The Finger Slide

Place your hand flat, fingers spread, on the table. Lift and slide each finger toward the thumb. Resist slightly with the other hand. This will help prevent drifting of the fingers toward the little-finger side of the hand.

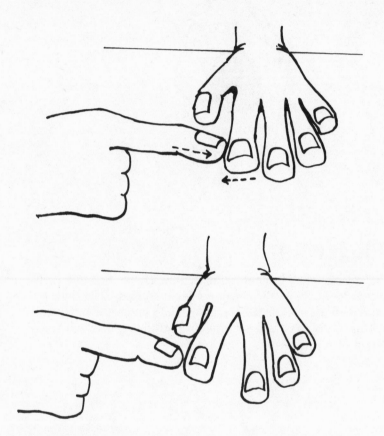

WRISTS

37. The Wrist Press

This exercise will strengthen the muscles that bend and straighten the wrist. Rest your hand on a table or armrest. Place the heel of the other hand on top. Raise the bottom hand, pushing against the top hand. Hold for six seconds, then relax. Reverse positions of the hand and repeat. Remember, while you are pressing the hands together, allow no joint movement. If it is painful to use your other hand as the stationary object, try to lift the hand against another stable object, such as the chair arm.

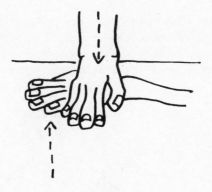

ELBOWS

38. The Biceps Bulge

This will strengthen the muscles that bend and straighten the elbow. Place your exercise belt slightly above each wrist, palms facing up. Bend one elbow and straighten the other, pulling the belt tight. Hold for six seconds. Relax. Reverse arm positions. If you do not have an exercise belt, cross your forearms, palms up, and press together. Hold for six seconds. Relax and reverse arm positions.

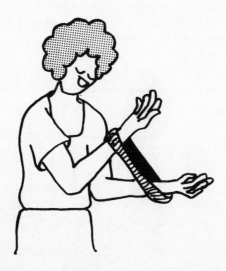

SHOULDERS

39. The Side Pull

Place the exercise belt around your forearms. With the elbows straight, palms facing each other, move your arms out to the side until the belt is tight. Hold for six seconds. Relax. If you do not have an exercise belt, perform the same movement, pushing against a wall, door frame, or some other stationary object.

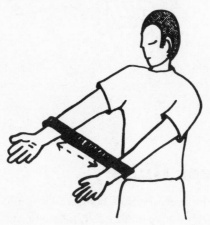

40. The Robot

This exercise will strengthen the muscles that raise and lower your arm. Place the exercise belt around your forearms, palms down. Keeping elbows straight, pull up with one arm and down with the other until the belt is tight. Hold for six seconds, then relax. Reverse arm positions and repeat. If you do not have an exercise belt, perform the same movement using a table, wall, or your other forearm as the stationary object.

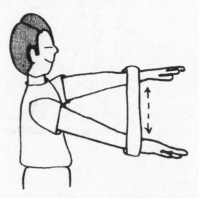

41. The Bow and Arrow

This is a fun exercise for strengthening many of the arm muscles. Hold the exercise belt in both hands. Push out to the side with one arm and pull back with the other, as if shooting a bow and arrow or a giant rubber band. Hold for six seconds, then relax. Reverse arm positions. Those with hand involvement should modify this exercise because gripping the belt causes stress. Be creative!

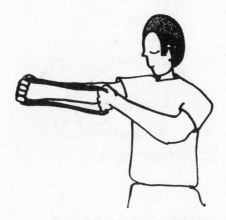

HIPS

42. The "Cheek to Cheek"

This exercise will strengthen the muscles that move your leg backward. Squeeze the buttocks tightly together. Hold for six seconds. Relax. This exercise may be done while lying down, sitting, or standing.

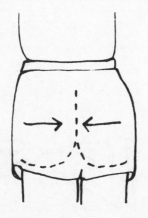

43. The Leg Spreader

The muscles that move your legs out to the side must be strong if you are to walk well. Lie on your back, with the exercise belt placed around your ankles. (If your knees are painful place the belt above the knees.) Spread your legs apart until the exercise belt is as tight as possible. Hold for six seconds, then relax. Do not let your foot roll in or out. You may do each leg separately if you wish.

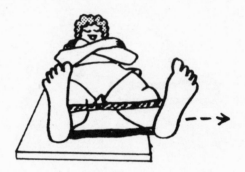

44. The Straight-Leg Raise

This familiar old exercise will strengthen the muscles that bend the hip as well as the muscle that runs across the front of the knee. Lie on your back, arms in a comfortable position. Tighten the muscle that runs across the front of the knee and then raise your leg one to two feet off the ground, keeping the knee straight. Do not arch your back. Hold for six seconds. Relax. If you have low back discomfort you should do this exercise with the other knee bent. As your muscles become stronger, place the exercise belt around your ankles and perform the same exercise. Pull the belt tight, hold for six seconds, and then lower the leg slowly.

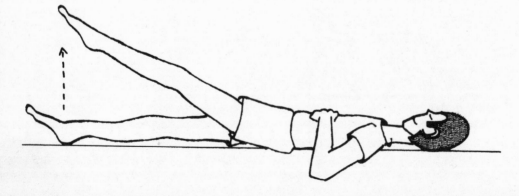

KNEES

45. The Quad Set

This is a good place for the person with very weak or painful knees to start. The exercise will strengthen the muscles that straighten the knee. These muscles are crucial for walking, going up and down stairs, or getting out of low furniture. Sit with your back supported, legs stretched out in front of you. (You may bend one knee if this is more comfortable.) Tighten the muscle that runs across the front of the knee by pulling your toes toward your head and pushing the back of the knee down into the bed or floor. Hold for six seconds. Relax. If sitting is difficult, this exercise may be done while lying down.

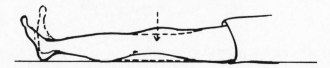

46. The Knee Scissor

Here's another exercise to strengthen the muscles that straighten the knee. It will also strengthen the muscles that bend the knee. Sit in a straight-backed chair. Place the exercise belt around both ankles. Straighten one knee while you pull back with the other until the belt is very tight. Hold for six seconds. Relax. To reduce stress on the knee joint, lean back slightly as you do this exercise.

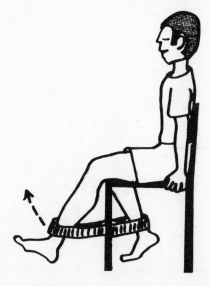

47. The Heel Press

To strengthen the muscles at the back of the thigh that bend the knee, sit in a straight-backed chair. Bend the knee, pressing the heel against the leg of the chair. Hold for six seconds. Relax.

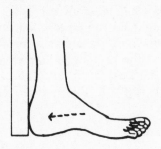

ANKLES AND FEET

48. The Tiptoe

Holding on lightly to a counter or table for support, raise up on your tiptoes (A).

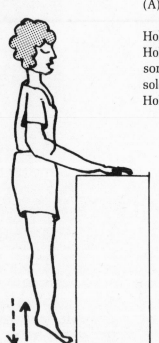

Holding on lightly to a counter or table for support, raise up on your tiptoes (A). Hold for six seconds. Lower slowly. This exercise may be too stressful for some, especially if you are overweight. As an alternative exercise, place the sole of your foot against a stationary object (wall, chair leg) and push (B). Hold for six seconds; relax.

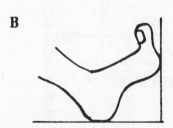

NECK

If your neck pain is a new occurrence and the pain is moderate to severe, if you have pain that radiates down your arm with neck movement, or if numbness, tingling, or marked weakness are present in the arm, consult a doctor or physiotherapist before proceeding with these exercises.

49. The Head Press

Here is an easy way to strengthen the muscles that bend and straighten the neck. Place your forearm against your forehead and press with your head. Hold for six seconds, allowing no movement. Relax. Then place your forearm on the back of the head and push. Hold for six seconds. Relax. If you cannot use your arm as the stationary object, a wall or a car headrest will do just as well.

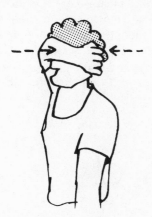 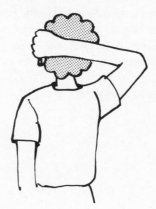

50. The Neck Strengthener

The same muscles can be strengthened while lying in bed. Lift your head up off the pillow. Hold for six seconds, then relax. Press your head down into the pillow. Hold for six seconds, then relax. If lifting your head is painful, press against your forearm as in exercise 49.

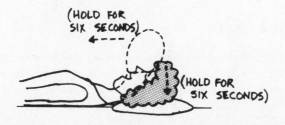

BACK AND STOMACH

If your back pain is a new occurrence and the pain is moderate to severe, if pain radiates down your leg or around to the chest, or if numbness, tingling, or marked weakness exist, consult a doctor or physiotherapist before proceeding.

Firm stomach and back muscles are important to provide the support necessary for an erect posture and to avoid back strain. In addition to the following exercises, the Pelvic Tilt (exercise 28) is helpful and should be done frequently during the day, in any position.

51. The Partial Sit-Up

It is not necessary to do a full sit-up to exercise the stomach muscles. A partial sit-up will place less stress on the joints and is sufficient. Lie on your back on a firm surface, knees bent, feet flat. Raise your head and shoulders as far off the surface as possible. Hold for six seconds, then lower slowly. Breathe out as you raise your body, count to six out loud as you hold, and breathe in as you lower your body. *Do not hold your breath.* If your neck is painful during this exercise, try the next one instead. Don't cheat by tucking your feet under a chair!

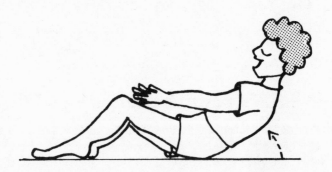

52. The Back Sit

This is a fun alternative to the sit-up and is easier on the neck. Sit upright on a firm surface. Lean partially backward, hold for six seconds, then return to sitting. As your stomach muscles strengthen you should be able to lean farther and farther backward. Breathe out as you lean back, count to six out loud as you hold, and breathe in as you return to sitting.

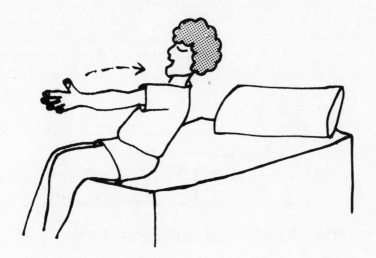

53. The Back Push

To strengthen the muscles that straighten the back, sit in a straight-backed chair or against the wall. Push your shoulders and shoulder blades into the chair or wall. Hold for six seconds. Relax. You will feel the stomach muscles tighten as well; the stomach muscles help support the back.

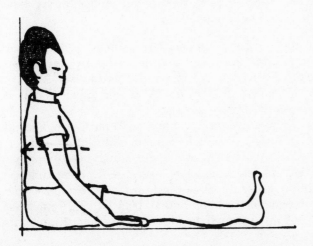

54. The Back Lift

This exercise will also strengthen the muscles that straighten the back, but it is more strenuous. Lie on your stomach, arms at your sides. Lift your head, shoulders, and arms up off the floor or bed. Hold for six seconds. Relax. If this does not feel too stressful, try lifting your legs off the floor at the same time. This is generally not a good exercise for the person with moderate to severe low back pain but is beneficial for the person with general stiffness or ankylosing spondylitis.

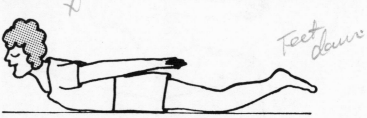

A MATTER OF PRINCIPLE: EXERCISE REVIEW

Let's go back over the critical points. The two most important kinds of exercise to maintain and improve the function of arthritic joints and surrounding muscles are:

1. **Stretching exercises** to maintain and increase joint mobility and thus function. They should be performed three to ten times a session, two to four times a day, depending on pain.

2. **Strengthening exercises** to increase muscle strength and improve the ability to bear weight, lift objects, and sustain movement. Usually, isometric exercises are best. Hold each exercise for six seconds and repeat three to four times once a day.

Endurance and relaxation activities should also be a part of your daily schedule to provide for a well-rounded exercise programme. Balance your exercise activities with times of rest during the day. You can combine rest periods with relaxation training. Also remember that it is important to prepare for exercise by warming up.

Design your own exercise programme to meet your special needs. Assess each exercise for its benefit to your priority joints and for any excessive stress on other involved joints. Begin slowly and build your programme according to your response to the exercise. If at any time exercise-induced pain continues for more than two hours after exercise, you are doing too much. Do not stop exercising, but cut back a little. Remember, if you have a hot joint, restrain yourself to moving the joint through its full range of motion twice a day.

A MATTER OF PROGRAMME: SETTING UP YOUR OWN EXERCISE PROGRAMME

Now that you have chosen specific exercises, it may be helpful to write out your exercise programme and keep an exercise diary. This tends to help you get started, and when you look back on it, it will show you how far you have progressed.

GUIDELINES

The following will give you some guidelines for setting up your exercise programme. Read these guidelines carefully and use them as you plan your programme.

Stretching Exercises (Exercises 1-33)

1. Start doing three repetitions of each exercise twice a day.

2. If for four days you have no exercise-induced pain lasting longer than two hours, add two repetitions (five in all) and do the exercises three times a day.

3. If no exercise-induced pain lasting longer than two hours is present in an additional four-day period, add two more repetitions (seven in all) and do the exercises four times a day.

4. If in the next four days you have no exercise-induced pain lasting longer than two hours, add three more repetitions (ten in all) and do the exercises four times a day.

5. If exercise-induced pain continues for more than two hours after exercise, cut back to the next lowest level and continue at that level for four days, then try the next highest level again.

6. If exercise-induced pain lasting longer than two hours occurs at the first level, try not to stretch so far (just past the point of pain). If pain still persists, cut back to two repetitions once a day or choose a different exercise that will achieve the same result.

7. Once you have reached your goal for a joint, remember to move it through its maximum range at least once or twice a day. This will ensure that you maintain the mobility that you worked so hard to obtain. If you notice that you are losing ground with that joint, then resume a more concentrated exercise programme.

Strengthening Exercises (Exercises 34-54)

1. Start doing each exercise twice, once a day.

2. If no exercise-induced pain lasting longer than two hours occurs in a four-day period, add one repetition (three in all).

3. If no exercise-induced pain occurs for four more days, add one repetition (four in all).

4. If exercise-induced pain continues for more than two hours after exercise, cut back to the next lowest level and continue at that level for four days, then try to move to the next highest level again.

5. If pain occurs at the first level, reduce the force of your exercise. If pain still persists, cut back to doing the exercise only once.

Now write your own initial programme and follow your progress using the exercise diary.

EXERCISE DIARY   Week of _____

Day	Figure Number	Number of Repetitions	Times a Day	Pain

6
Protecting Your Joints

Joint protection plays an important role in the management of arthritis, especially in rheumatoid arthritis. Because of inflammation or instability, arthritic joints may be unable to withstand the stresses applied during normal daily activities. Forces imposed from such simple activities as opening the car door, turning on the tap, or climbing stairs may cause increased pain levels and may contribute to joint deterioration.

Joint protection is a means of using your joints wisely. In a broad sense, this entire book is about protecting your joints. Taking the appropriate medication, exercising your joints to their full range and strength, and eating a well-balanced diet are all ways of ensuring maximum joint function.

There are, however, some very specific principles that may be beneficial for your individual needs. These principles will help you to attain the three main goals of joint protection: (1) minimizing stress and pain, (2) maintaining mobility and function, and (3) conserving your energy.

MINIMIZING JOINT STRESS AND PAIN

What produces stress on a joint? Joint stress comes from factors such as time and force and depends on the type of arthritis. Strong forces over a short period of time or mild forces over long periods of time can contribute to further joint damage. For the arms and hands, a stressful force may occur during activities involving squeezing, pushing, pulling, twisting, and lifting movements. The weight-bearing joints—hips, knees, ankles, and feet—can be overstressed from either excessive body weight or activities that place increased loads on these joints. For example, walking on a level surface may not be bothersome, but getting up from a chair, climbing stairs, jogging, and carrying two grocery bags "load" these joints with more than body weight. The spine—back and neck—can be stressed by bending over, twisting while reaching for an object, and poor standing, sitting, or sleeping postures.

Overstressing a joint can contribute to intensified pain. In fact, the most common sign of joint stress is pain. Activity-induced pain is thus a warning sign for you to take it easier on that joint.

A painful joint is in many ways like a strained muscle. If in the initial stages of recovery the muscle is subjected to more activity than it can tolerate, the muscle will be more painful and will take longer to heal. On the other hand, a certain amount of movement by the muscle will facilitate the healing process. Optimum function for both the joint and the muscle is achieved by using the appropriate type and amount of activity. Both this joint protection and the exercise sections will assist you in determining the proper type and amount of activity for you.

Severe pain during a specific task or increased pain lasting for one to two hours after an activity should alert you to start the following steps:

1. Be aware of your body. Learn to recognize activity-induced pain.

2. Determine the particular movements that cause pain.

3. Use principles of joint protection to change the method of performing the activity.

The following principles are subdivided by the specific joints to which they apply. Select the principles that match your problem areas. Since learning new habits or new movement patterns takes time, begin by working with only one or two principles. As they are mastered, begin to incorporate additional principles into your daily routine.

PRINCIPLE 1   For Hands, Arms, and Back
Use the strongest or largest joint possible to accomplish a task.

This means that instead of using your fingers, use the palm of your hand, your forearm, or your elbow; instead of your arms, use your whole body; instead of your back, use your legs. In this way, the stress is distributed over the largest area possible. The larger the area, the more pressure, weight, and/or force the joint can tolerate.

Examples
Fingers

Spare your hands from difficult-to-open refrigerator doors or cupboards by placing a strap on the handle. To open, simply place your forearm through the strap and pull.

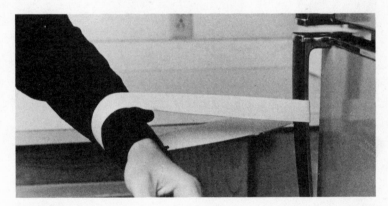

A doorknob extender allows you to open the door with the palm of the hand instead of with the fingers.

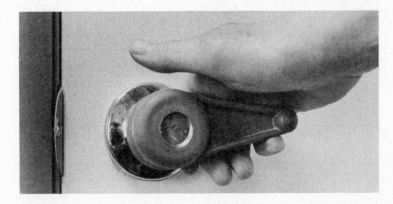

Hands and Elbows

Carry a purse on your forearm or use a shoulder bag to avoid clutching in your hand.

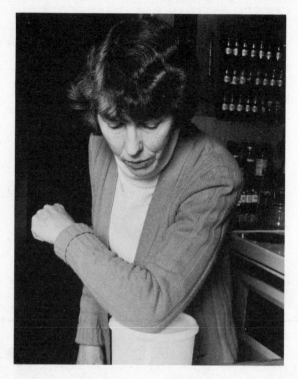

Close plastic containers with your elbow.

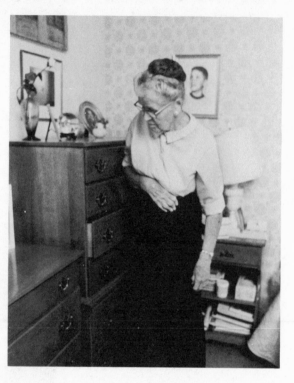

Use your hip to close kitchen or dresser drawers.

Back

To lift heavy objects from the floor, bend your knees instead of the back.

PRINCIPLE 2   For the Hands, Arms, and Knees
Distribute the load over several joints.

This can often be accomplished by using both arms together to lift, push, or pull objects. The concept is similar to principle 1, except that you want to distribute the stress over as many joints as possible.

Examples
Hands and Arms

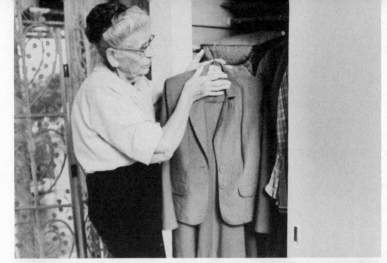

Use both arms to take down or hang clothes in the wardrobe.

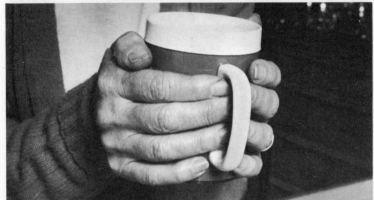

Instead of placing your fingers through the handle, encircle a coffee cup with both hands. Mugs are especially good for this.

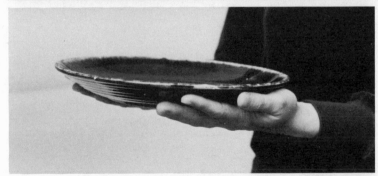

Carry your plate back to the kitchen by "scooping" it up with the palms of both hands.

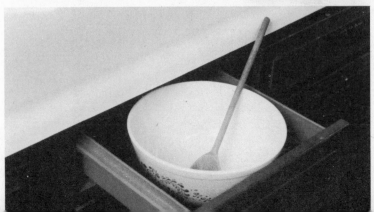

Use both hands to mix or stir by wedging the bowl in a drawer. Even better, of course, would be to use an electric mixer.

Examples

Knees

Sit in chairs with armrests so that you may push with your arms to stand up.

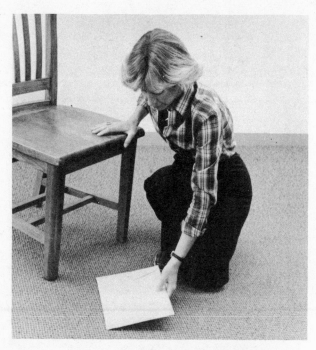

When stooping down to reach an object, use the edge of a chair or table to push up. (If your wrists or elbows are involved, however, you probably should avoid this because they may receive too much stress from your body weight.)

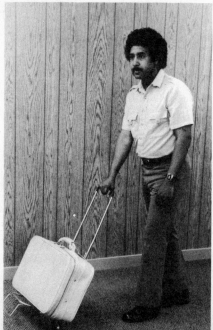

Use a luggage carrier when traveling. This allows you to take most of the strain off your arms as you push or pull the suitcase.

PRINCIPLE 3　For Hands, Arms, Knees, and Back

Use each joint in its most stable and functional position.

Each joint has a range in which it is most stable and from which it can work most effectively. This range is determined not only by the structure of the joint, but also by the muscles of the joint. Certain positions will allow for greater leverage and maximum efficiency of the muscles. These are usually positions where the joint is in a straight alignment, not bent or rotated to the side.

Examples

Knees

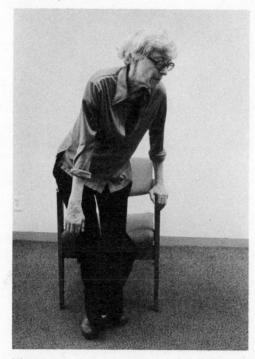
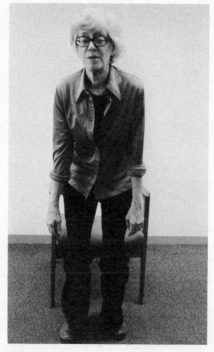

Wrong　　　　　　　　　　　　　　　　Right

When standing up, keep both feet flat on the floor and pointed ahead. Stand straight up. Avoid pushing with one hand to prevent leaning to one side, causing harmful twisting strains on the knees.

Back

When opening a drawer, cupboard, or door, position yourself directly in front of it to prevent twisting of the trunk.

To pick up an object, make sure you face it directly, again to avoid twisting the trunk.

Hands

The position of your hand in relation to your forearm will determine the strength of your grip. Keep the hand in a straight alignment with the arm and bend the wrist backward slightly during most activities.

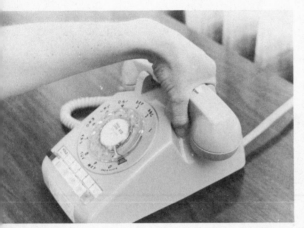

Wrong

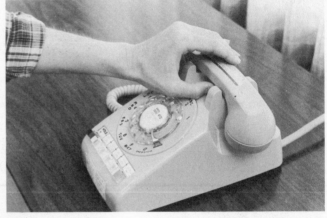

Right

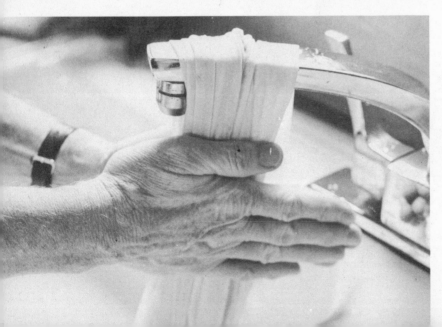

Wringing out wet washcloths or laundry places twisting motions on top of the strong pressures involved in squeezing. Wrap the item over the tap and squeeze excess water out between the palms of your hands. An alternative is to wrap the item in a thick towel and let the towel soak up the excess moisture.

PRINCIPLE 4   Mostly for the Back and Neck
Use good body mechanics.

Body mechanics refers to the development of good posture and movement habits during daily activities. A key component of posture is the Pelvic Tilt, described earlier in the exercise section of Chapter 6 (exercise 28). The degree that the pelvis is tilted in relation to the spine helps determine how straight the spine is aligned. The better the alignment, the less strain on both muscles and joints.

 To feel this position, please refer to exercise 28 on page 46. While doing these exercises, focus your awareness on the trunk and hips and try to maintain this position, the pelvic tilt, later during the day.

Examples
Standing

When standing for prolonged periods of time is necessary, alternate your positions between the following:

Wrong   **Right**

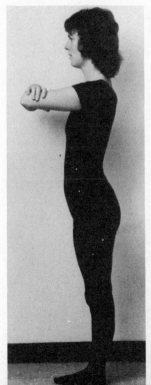 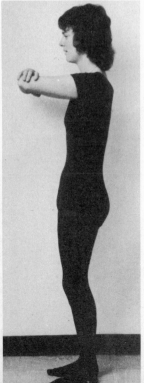

Stand with weight distributed equally between both feet. For a back problem, to assist with maintaining the pelvic tilt, avoid locking your knees. Don't do this if you also have a knee problem.

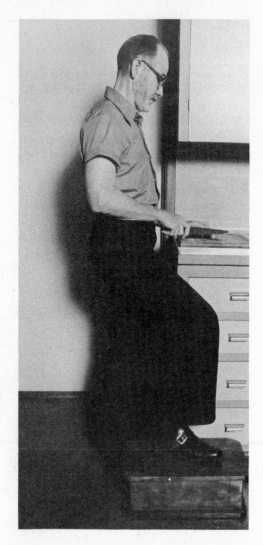

Place one foot on a footstool. This helps to maintain a pelvic tilt and thus alleviate low back strain.

Wear flat or low-heeled shoes, not only for the greater stability and safety they afford, but also because they help to keep the pelvis tilted.

Sitting

Select chairs that provide adequate support for your back. A firm seat and fairly straight back will help you to avoid slouching.

When writing at a desk, do not lean forward, but sit tall and bend the neck only slightly.

Persons with neck problems may want to consider a drafting table with an adjustable slant.

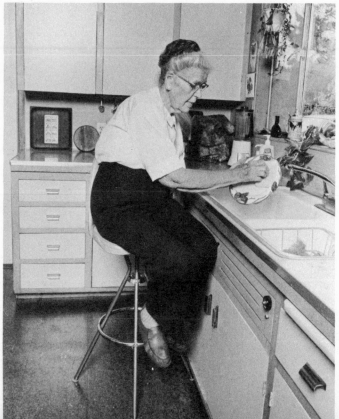

When working at your workbench or in the kitchen, a bar-height stool with footrest allows you to half-sit, half-stand. This helps to prevent fatigue, as well as to provide a suitable height for working on projects, washing dishes, or preparing meals.

Standing Up

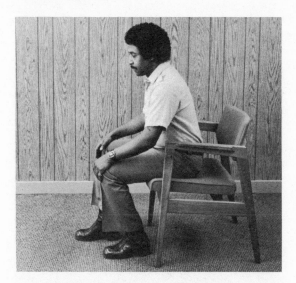

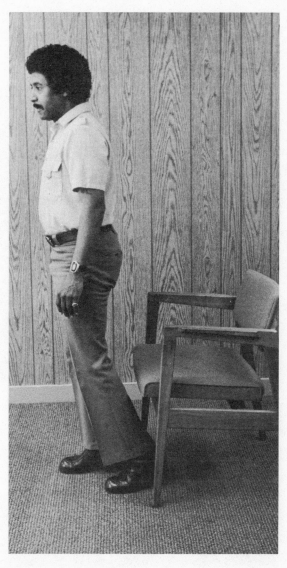

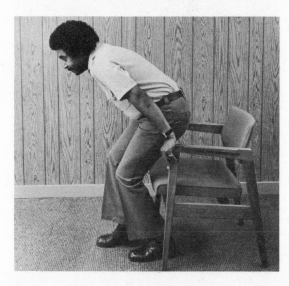

The most efficient method, utilizing good body mechanics and thus less muscle power, requires that you plan ahead. First, shuffle forward in your chair so that you are near the edge. Second, place one foot slightly in front of the other so that it is directly under the knee. The other foot is behind the knee. Then lean forward until your hips automatically start to come off the chair.

Chairs that are several inches higher than normal, either through the use of pillows or chair leg extenders, make it easier to stand up.

Lifting

To lift objects from the ground or low shelves, bend your legs instead of your back; pick up the object, holding it as close to your body as possible, and rise, letting your leg muscles do the work.

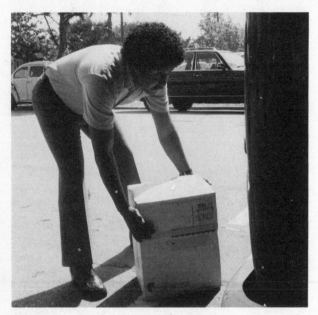

Wrong

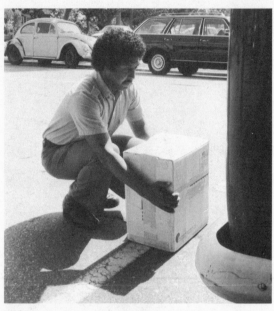

Right

Persons with knee involvement may want to let someone else lift heavy objects, since the knees will be strained from the weight of the object as well as from their own body weight.

PRINCIPLE 5
Reduce the effort required to do the job.

There are various ways to reduce the amount of effort we exert. In fact, all of the principles mentioned above involve this to some degree. However, there are some additional concepts that provide ways to modify either the tools or the activity itself.

These include: (1) using adaptive devices or tools suitable to the task, (2) employing leverage, and (3) avoiding lifting and carrying.

Examples

Use adaptive devices.

There are various aids or devices that have been developed for the express purpose of alleviating joint stress and pain. Others were developed to simplify all of our lives in one way or another, but they also act to protect joints. Some of these can be found in department or economy stores; others are available through either occupational therapy departments or special catalogues. Information can be obtained from Arthritis Care.

Examples of adaptive devices are illustrated at various points in this chapter, as well as in Chapter 7. The main point is that although it is not generally recommended that you accumulate a huge number of gadgets, it is important to make use of devices that will protect your joints. An occupational therapist can assist you in determining your equipment needs.

Employ leverage.

A piece of wood, metal, or firm plastic can be attached to many types of objects to increase the area for gripping. The longer the attachment or lever, the less pressure required to manipulate the desired object.

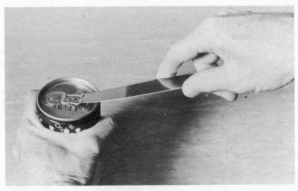

Open ring or flip-top cans with a knife.

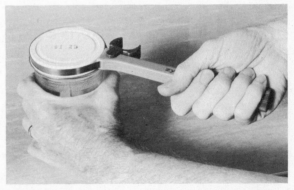

Certain types of jar openers are constructed with a long handle, thus employing the principle of leverage.

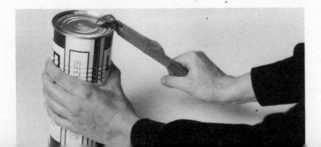

Attach a dowel or a piece of wood to a can opener and hold onto this lengthened handle when opening cans.

Avoid lifting and carrying.

Slide or push objects.

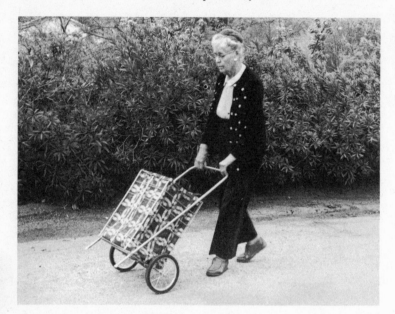

Use wheels to transport. Trolleys, tea tables, and shopping trolleys are just a few examples of readily available items on wheels.

Wheels attached to your dustbin, either permanently or in the form of a small trolley which holds the bin, save lifting a heavy weight.

MAINTAINING JOINT MOBILITY AND FUNCTION

The minimizing of joint stress and pain discussed above ties in directly with mobility and function. In the absence of pain, we are able to move our bodies freely—our bodies function well. When we experience pain, however, our natural reaction is to try to reduce it. Unfortunately, this is often accomplished by limiting movement and by keeping the affected joint in a bent position. This can produce a vicious cycle in which pain leads to an unwillingness to move, stiffness and shortening of muscles and joint tissues result, and there is a further increase in pain and difficulty with movement.

While minimizing pain is a crucial aspect of joint protection, one must be careful not to sacrifice mobility.

Wrong: disease ⟶ dis-use ⟶ dys-function

Right: dis-ease ⟶ proper use ⟶ maintain function

There are times, of course, when activities need to be limited. The rules for exercising a hot joint are applicable to activities. At these times, activities involving free and easy motions with little resistance are to be encouraged, while activities with resistance should be avoided. As the inflammation subsides, gradually work back to your normal level of activity.

PRINCIPLE 6   For Hips, Knees, Ankles, and Hands

Avoid prolonged periods of maintaining the same joint position.

There are two main points that illustrate the importance of this rule. First, joints affected by arthritis have a tendency to stiffen. Therefore, frequent position changes are essential to maintain mobility. Second, muscles that are fixed or tensed will fatigue. Fatigued muscles are not able to provide adequate support for your joints.

Examples

Hips and Knees

Alternate between sitting and standing positions. Although the sitting position is generally recommended to reduce stress on the lower joints and prevent fatigue, it is important to get up and stretch frequently.

Knees

When sitting, change the position of your legs so that your knees are often stretched out, feet supported by a footstool.

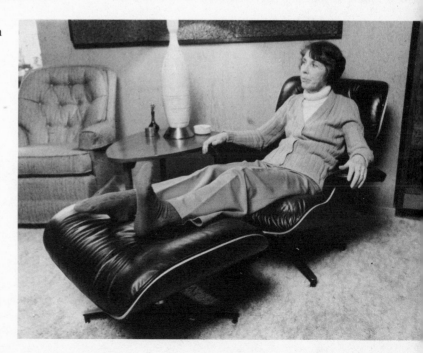

Ankles

Bend and point your toes while watching television or talking with a friend. You don't have to wait for a specific exercise time to do your range-of-motion exercises.

Hands

Avoid sustained grasps on objects. For example, instead of writing with a pen, use a typewriter.

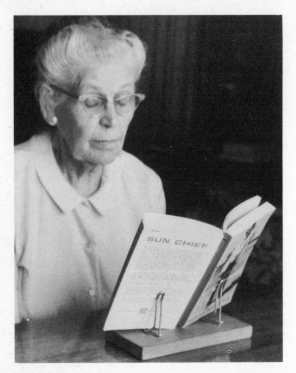 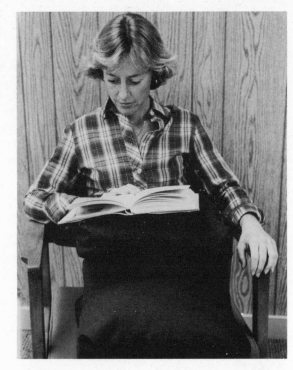

A book holder or pillows on your lap will serve as a means to support a book and will free your hands.

When it is necessary to maintain your grasp on an object for more than several minutes, take frequent breaks to stretch and move your fingers.

PRINCIPLE 7 For Arms

Encourage full and complete motions during daily activities.

Many daily activities, when performed correctly, provide movement patterns that can serve as an adjunct to your regular exercise programme. They can stretch and strengthen. For example, long, sweeping, flowing strokes can help to maintain and increase the range of motion of a joint.

Examples

Shoulders

When ironing, straighten the arm as far as possible, using long, flowing strokes.

To vacuum, use a long, forward stroke with the vacuum, then pull it in close to the body so the arm is first fully straightened, then fully bent. If you have elbow or shoulder pain, however, you want to either walk with the vacuum cleaner as you move it forward or purchase the lightest model possible.

Encourage shoulder mobility by placing light objects on high shelves where you will have to reach to get them.

Reach as high as possible when washing windows.

PRINCIPLE 8 Primarily for the Knees, Arms, and Hands

Avoid positions and activities leading to possible joint deformities.

Deformities occur more frequently in rheumatoid arthritis than in any other kind of arthritis. Long-term disease may produce changes in joint structure, with consequent limitations of movement. When joint motion is limited, daily activities become difficult or, in some cases, impossible to perform.

As mentioned earlier, joints tend to be held in flexed or bent positions for comfort, which is a primary reason that deformities occur. Move out of such positions frequently. The following are examples of more appropriate postures.

Examples

Knees

Sleeping with pillows under the knees should be avoided unless otherwise advised.

When sitting, place your legs on a footrest to keep your knees straight for part of the time.

Elbows

Stretch your arms out in front of you or by your side when sitting or lying.

Hands

The hands, which contain intricate mechanisms, are prone to damage. The most common hand deformities of rheumatoid arthritis are swan's neck, ulnar deviation, and boutonniere.

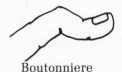

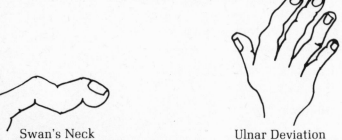

Swan's Neck   Ulnar Deviation   Boutonniere

There are several procedures to help prevent these deformities. These are reviewed below; however, consultation with an occupational therapist is recommended if you are beginning to develop these problems. The two sub-principles are:

PRINCIPLE 8A
Avoid excessive pressure against the back of the fingers, the pads of the thumb and fingers, and the thumb side of each finger.

Examples

The Back of the Fingers

When pushing up from a chair, keep your hands facing palm down.

Wrong

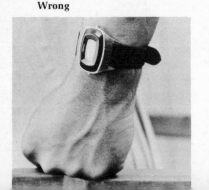

Right

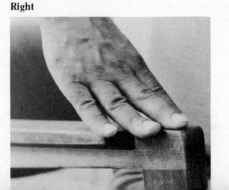

Right

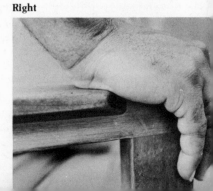

If you prop your chin in your hand, keep the palm of the hand toward your face.

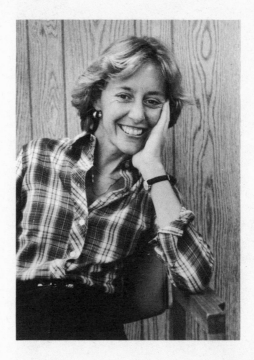

Right

The Pads of the Thumb and Fingers

When using spray cans or bottles, push down with the palm of the hand instead of the thumbtip.

Wrong   **Right**

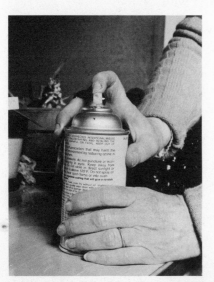

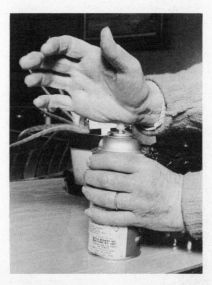

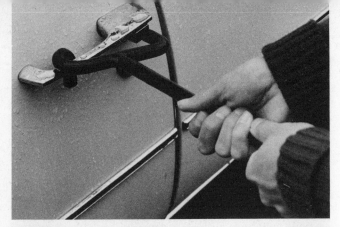

Open a car door with an aid in the palm of your hand.

Never use a butterfly can opener, because the pressure required to operate these is extreme; use an electric or wall-mounted type.

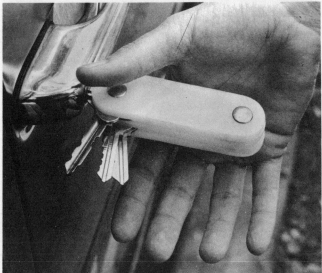

Special key holder devices allow you to turn a key by holding the handle in the palm of your hand. These are available through special-equipment firms or can be made by riveting a piece of wood or metal to the key.

The Thumb Side of Each Finger

To prevent ulnar deviation, turn jar lids, taps, and doorknobs *toward* the thumb. This means that doors should be opened with the left hand and jars with the right.

Perform activities involving circular motions such as stirring, dusting, and washing dishes *toward* the thumb side of the hand. This is a counterclockwise motion with the right hand and clockwise with the left.

Use a wire-brush scourer with a handle to clean pots and pans. This allows you to hold the scourer in the palm of the hand instead of with the fingertips.

Try writing with the pencil held between the index and middle fingers.

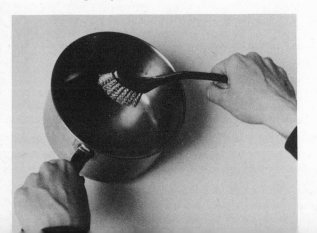

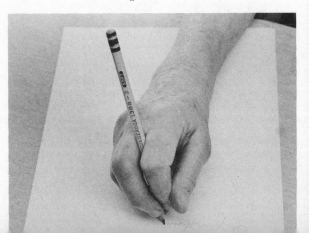

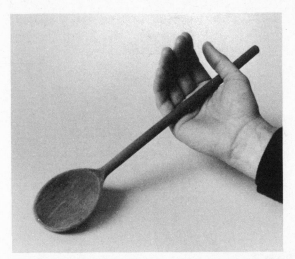 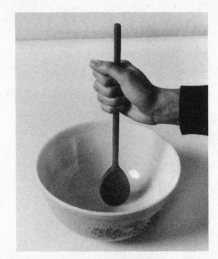

Use a cylindrical grasp on objects with handles; place the handle parallel to the knuckles. This includes such objects as mixing spoons, knives, tools, and brooms.

PRINCIPLE 8B

Avoid tight grasps on objects and keep hands open whenever possible.

Examples

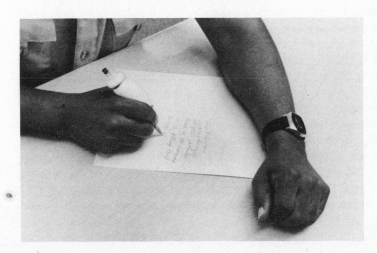

Foam padding added to such articles as a toothbrush, pen, razor, fork, and comb will increase the size of the handle. The larger the grip, the less tension required to maintain your hold on these objects.

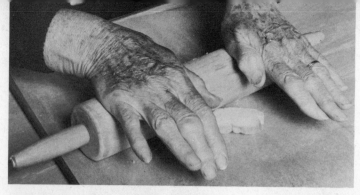

Instead of holding onto the handles of a rolling pin, place hands flat on top and roll beneath your hands.

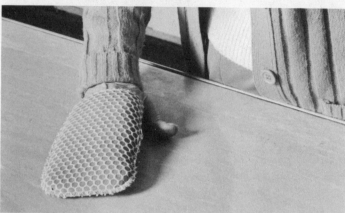

To wash dishes, there is a scrubber that fits over your hand available in supermarkets or hardware stores. Since you don't need to grasp it, you can keep your fingers in a straightened position.

Use a sponge instead of a dishrag to mop up tables and counters. The water can be squeezed out of the sponge more easily by putting it in the sink and pressing down with your flattened hand.

CONSERVING YOUR ENERGY

Did you conserve energy today? This question does not refer to natural resources such as gas and coal, but to your own body and its energy expenditures. A great deal of energy is expended unnecessarily by each of us in the normal course of the day. And just as natural resources are not easily replenished, neither are our own. If we work for several hours or a full day, we often don't have the energy in the evening to do more than collapse in front of the television. It would be nice to be able to pursue hobbies and other interests with as much energy as we felt earlier in the day.

Energy conservation techniques benefit all of us. Although much of it is simply common sense, energy conservation is actually a science that evolved from the desire to conserve energy and increase efficiency. Energy conservation techniques are particularly important for certain types of arthritis (notably rheumatoid), since feelings of fatigue and lethargy often accompany these diseases. In addition, energy conservation acts to protect joints by using your body efficiently, thus minimizing muscle fatigue, joint stress, and pain.

Several of the principles of energy conservation are briefly described below.

PRINCIPLE 9
Organize your work.

Each individual task, as well as each workday, can be organized ahead of time to prevent wasted time and motion. Try to get the most done with the least amount of effort.

Examples

"Think before you act." Develop your planning and organizing skills by starting with a pencil and paper and writing lists. Identify what needs to get done and in what order of importance. Focus on one or more particular tasks.

Combine several errands in one trip whenever possible. If you have to go upstairs or to another part of the house or place of work, try to accomplish several things at a time.

Plan for an easy flow of work by storing equipment and supplies where they will be used first; for example, keep pots for cooking vegetables near the sink or the stove.

Avoid rush by planning ahead. Hasty movements are often no more quickly accomplished than planned, purposeful movements, and they often end in extra work, as with the old adage, "Haste makes waste." Both tension and fatigue are increased when we feel rushed.

PRINCIPLE 10
Balance work with rest.

One of the most effective means of avoiding fatigue is to schedule short but frequent rest periods throughout the day. Resting before you get tired is often difficult because we all want to get our work done. If we can prevent fatigue, even if it means stopping in the middle of a job, our endurance over the long run will be increased. When stopping to rest is difficult to do, remember that long work periods require longer recovery periods.

Examples

Schedule frequent rest periods throughout the day. This will vary for each individual, but an example might be to rest ten minutes out of every hour, instead of working for three hours straight.

Alternate heavy and light work tasks during each day. In addition, plan the more difficult or lengthy tasks when you know you have the endurance to complete them.

Sitting to work is a form of rest since it uses less energy than standing. However, if you spend your workday behind a desk, you will find that moving around at regular intervals will help to keep you more alert and energetic.

PRINCIPLE 11
Use efficient storage.

Efficient storage arrangements will help to (1) reduce the number of steps you take to gather all the necessary supplies and (2) minimize bending, stooping, and needless searching in unorganized places.

Examples

Determine easy-to-reach areas and use them for the most frequently used supplies.

Store heavy items within easy reach, such as on countertops, and store lighter items on the higher or lower shelves.

Organize storage areas with dividers, special racks, turntables, and pull-out shelves. Many of these items are available in local stores or can be easily made by a carpenter.

Use pegboards and hooks to hang objects.

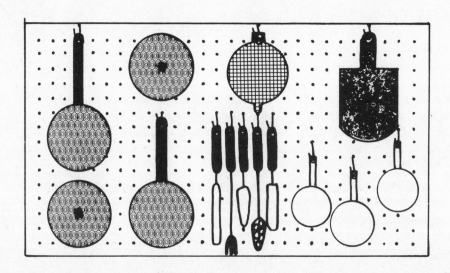

Have organized work centres for baking, clothes washing, hobbies, and so forth, where everything needed for a certain job is readily accessible. For example, a baking centre can be set up with the flour, sugar, and other spices kept in the same cupboard with the mixing bowls, measuring cups, and baking tins.

Remove unnecessary or infrequently used items from shelves.

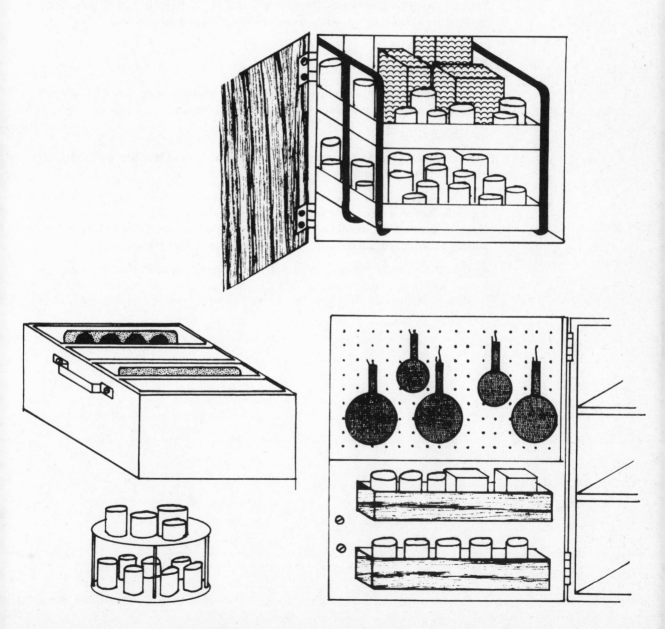

PRINCIPLE 12
Eliminate unnecessary tasks.

This is so self-explanatory it appears that no comments are necessary. "Voluntary simplicity" is a key to avoiding both stress and work.

Examples

If your homemaking standards for cleaning and cooking are higher than necessary, consider relaxing them to conserve energy.

Let dishes drip dry.

Use convenience foods or prepare foods in the easiest manner possible. For example, bake potatoes instead of mashing them.

Use the least amount of equipment possible. For example, measure the dry ingredients for a cake in a large two-cup measure and pour into the bowl. Next, measure and mix all the wet ingredients in the two-cup measure before adding to the dry ingredients. This eliminates an extra mixing bowl.

Realize that it is all right for you not to do everything and that you can ask family members to help you out. In fact, your family would probably prefer to lighten your load so that you can spend enjoyable, and not fatigued, time with them.

7
Self-Helpers
100 HINTS AND AIDS

The preceding chapter on joint protection provided you with basic principles and examples of how to protect your joints. Additional hints are provided in this chapter, not only on how to protect your joints, but also on how to do things if general mobility or finger coordination are impaired.

You may find that you already use many of the suggestions listed below. It is true that "necessity is the mother of invention." If you combine your needs and your common sense, you will probably come up with another 100 hints. Use these suggestions as a springboard for additional ideas to make your life easier and more comfortable. Then share them with friends and others who also could benefit from them.

DRESSING

If buttons are difficult to manipulate, sew Velcro on clothing, attach buttons permanently to the top side, and use the Velcro as a fastener. Velcro can be found in most sewing stores.

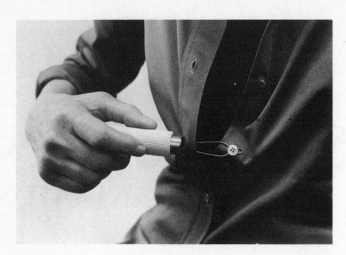

Buttonhooks work well to fasten buttons.

A final alternative for buttons on sleeves is to sew elasticized thread on button cuffs. This often provides sufficient give for your hands to slip through.

In the future, buy clothes that are easy to put on and easy to care for. Tops should be large enough or designed so that sleeves are easy to slip into—you may want to avoid turtlenecks. Elastic waistbands around trousers should be loose enough to slip easily over hips. Fastenings should be located in the front and be easy to manipulate.

If reaching the clothes in the wardrobe is difficult, have someone lower the rod.

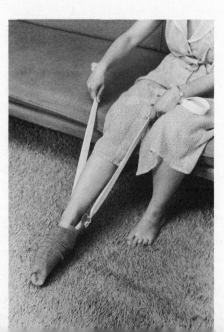

A stocking device will allow you to put socks on again if you can't reach your feet.

Special devices to assist with shoes include long-handled shoe horns, elastic shoelaces, and zipper laces.

A bent coat hanger, reacher, or dressing stick can assist with pulling trousers up, straightening shirts, or retrieving clothes slightly out of reach.

Place large rings or leather loops on zipper tabs.

BATHING AND HYGIENE

A long-handled sponge or brush can be used to soap yourself when bathing.

Tub and shower benches, or an old kitchen chair, can allow you to sit while bathing. This helps to prevent fatigue and provides a place to sit when getting down into the tub is difficult.

Safety considerations when bathing include the use of nonskid safety strips or a rubber bathmat on the floor. In addition, grab bars can be permanently installed on the wall or attached to the edge of the bathtub. Grab bars assist with safety when climbing in and out of the tub or shower and also provide a place to pull or push up from when in the tub.

A long shower spray hose makes rinsing easier.

After bathing, put on a terry robe and let it soak up the water as you pat yourself dry.

Use a shower caddy to keep soap and shampoo within easy reach.

Bath mitts can be bought or easily made by sewing two facecloths together. Lather it up and soap yourself the easy way.

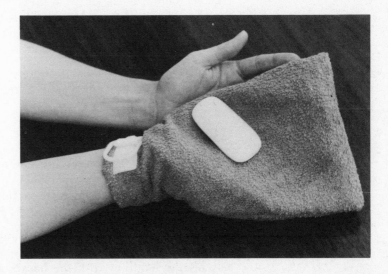

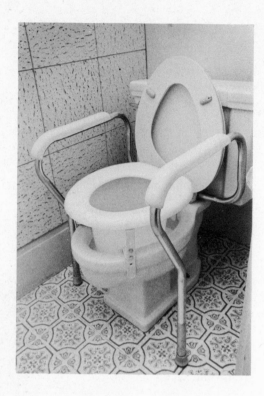

A raised toilet seat or commode over the toilet provides greater height and thus makes standing up easier.

In addition, a toilet safety frame or a grab bar installed in the wall next to the toilet will allow you to assist with your arms when sitting and standing.

Electric toothbrushes and Water-Piks make oral hygiene easier. In addition, there is a device that holds dental floss, allowing you to floss your teeth with one hand holding onto the handle—ask your dentist about this or check your local chemist.

Special long-handled combs and brushes are useful when shoulder and elbow limitations prevent reaching your head.

COOKING

Microwave ovens save time and energy. They are easy to operate, easy to clean, and easy to reach since they are usually placed on countertops. In addition, you do not need to worry about burning yourself since only the food heats up.

To avoid lifting pots heavy with food and the water it was boiled in, there are several alternatives. One is to place a frying basket inside a pot so that you may lift the food out with the basket and drain the water later. Spaghetti cookers come with a perforated insert and can serve in the same manner. Or you may want to ladle the contents out.

To open jars, install a jar opener that will grip the lid as you use both hands to turn the jar itself. Also, ask other members of the family not to close lids too tightly.

Use lightweight cooking utensils, bowls, and dishes. Avoid cast iron skillets and heavy ceramic bowls.

Select appliances with levers or push buttons that are easy to operate.

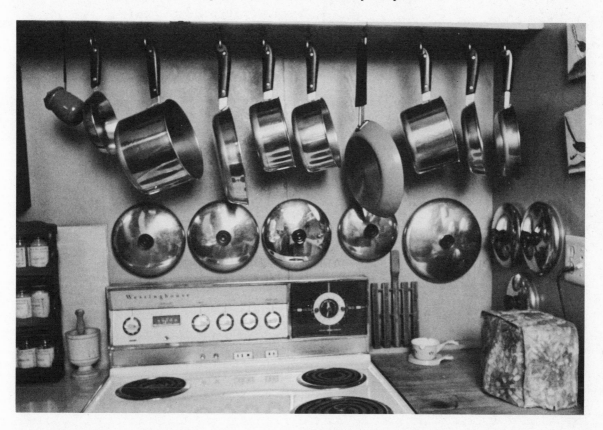

Use efficient storage arrangements. Have a "French kitchen" with pots, pans, and frequently used utensils hanging from the ceiling or wall fixtures.

Plan and prepare meals ahead of time to avoid last-minute preparations. Cook some meals the day before, let the flavors enhance, and then heat them up again the next day. Also, try preparing double or triple portions and freeze the extra.

Use biscuit tins and pans with special surfaces that prevent sticking and messy cleanup, or spray them with a nonstick product.

Mixing bowls can be stabilized by placing on a wet washcloth or on little octopus suction cups.

Place flour and sugar in containers so you can scoop out the amount needed and avoid lifting heavy bags each time.

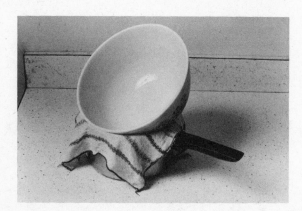

Use a pot with a wet cloth draped over it as a support for a bowl when pouring batter into a baking pan.

Mitt pot holders allow you to lift hot pans with the palms of both hands.

Use a bent coat hanger or dowel with a hook to pull oven shelves out when checking on the meal.

Attach a spray hose at the kitchen sink so that you can fill pots with water on the countertop; slide pots to the stove to avoid lifting.

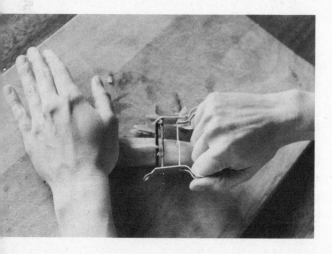

When peeling vegetables, try the kind of peeler with a handle you can slip your fingers through.

Instead of slicing onions, use an onion chopper.

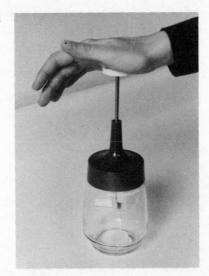

Try using a pizza wheel to cut various foods.

Food processors, the latest item to revolutionize the art of cooking, make food preparation easy, especially when large quantities of food must be chopped, sliced, or grated.

HOUSEKEEPING

Keep a set of cleaning supplies in each area where they are used to eliminate needless walking.

To clean the bathtub, sit on a low stool next to the tub and use a long-handled sponge.

Long-handled sponges can also be used to clean around door sills and other hard-to-reach places.

Use a long-handled dustpan and small broom to clean up dry spills from floors.

Use an adjustable-height ironing board so that you can sit to iron. Attach a cord-minder to keep the cord out of your way.

Carpeting or foam-backed rugs help to ease ankle and foot pain when prolonged standing and moving about are necessary.

Use gravity whenever possible. Let your clothes fall from the dryer into the basket. When scooping them out, you may want to use a reacher or stick.

Laundry bags that were originally intended for washing delicate items like nylons can be used for all small pieces of clothing (socks, underwear) and thus eliminate searching in the machine.

If lifting detergent boxes is difficult, you can either have someone else pour some into a smaller container or buy the bulk size and scoop it out. Liquid detergents may also be more manageable.

Try using the old-style push-on clothespegs rather than pinch clothespegs.

Front-loading washers are generally easier to use than top-loading washers. Raising the washer on blocks will also make laundering easier, since bending is eliminated.

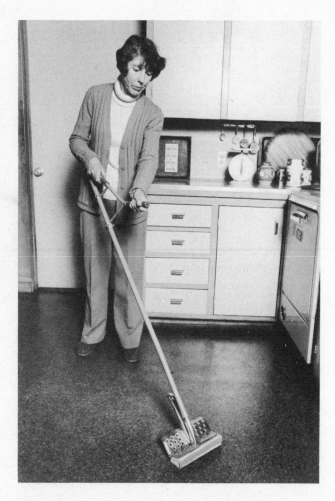

Use a Back Preserver tool on your floor mop or push broom. These tasks can be performed with better posture and less strain to the back with this special long-handled attachment.

If fitted sheets are difficult to manage, slit the last corner and fasten with a tie.

Use an oven shovel to tuck in sheets.

DRIVING

Auxiliary or wide-angle mirrors allow for increased visibility when neck movement is limited.

Special spinner knobs can be attached to the steering wheel to make steering easier when holding the wheel in the normal position is difficult.

To make driving more comfortable and to prevent low back strain, you may want to look into backrests, which are especially suitable for cars. They are similar to the cooling cushion inserts used when driving during the summer, but can be bent to fit your body curvatures and support your low back.

RECREATION OR LEISURE TIME

The best form of physical activity is swimming, since the buoyancy of the water helps to support the joints. In addition, much of your normal exercise routine can be performed while in the water. Check with the pools in your area to see if any of them provide "therapeutic pool" times, with water temperatures between 87 and 92 degrees.

An embroidery frame that can be attached to a table or chair will allow you to do needlework and sewing without using your hands to stabilize the article. These are available primarily through self-help aids catalogues.

If you like to play cards, try using a card holder. These can be purchased through mail-order catalogues or easily made by sawing a slit in a piece of wood.

If you enjoy gardening, there is now an attachment for spades. There is a different attachment to be used with hoes and rakes. These Back Preserver tools can easily be attached to your own equipment.

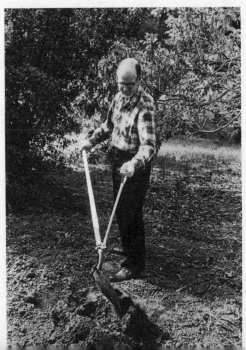

When gardening, try sitting on a small stool instead of kneeling to weed and plant.

Gardening can be made even easier by having a planter box or raised flower beds made. This will eliminate stooping entirely, as you can sit to work at a comfortable level.

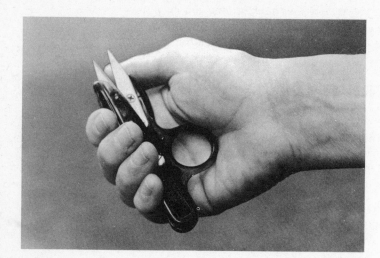

Use special clipping scissors when sewing to avoid pressure and pain on the thumb joint.

If threading a needle is difficult, self-threading needles or automatic threading machines are available through catalogues and in some sewing shops.

Afternoon exercises or sports are a really good way to break up the day. Try to set up a schedule at work where you can take an extended break to swim or exercise during the lunch hour.

JOINT WARM-UP (TO KEEP JOINTS WARM)

Use the extra-long heating pads that wrap around an arm or leg and fasten with Velcro to warm an elbow or knee.

Soak stiff, sore, or cold hands in warm water. This is especially useful to loosen them from morning stiffness. At night, warm the hands in this manner; rub hand lotion in and wear cotton gloves while sleeping.

Thermoelastic gloves are especially warming, since they are made from wool and elastic fibres. They are available in some chemist's.

Thermoelastic products are also available for knees and elbows. A soft, thick knee sock could also be used in the same manner. Cut the sock so you have a tube approximately seven inches long and place the tube over your knee or elbow.

Use electric blankets as a lightweight cover; they are especially useful in warming the bed before you get in it.

An alternative way to stay warm during the night or when resting is to sleep inside a sleeping bag that is placed under a blanket. The bag will turn with you and prevent cold air spaces.

Use a sleeping bag, cozy-wrap, or comforter when reading in a chair.

Use a mug to drink hot tea or coffee and hold it between both hands to warm them.

Slipper socks, worn over a pair of regular socks, will help to keep feet and ankles warm.

A new product on the market is the foot bath, which not only will warm your feet as they soak in the water but also can act as a massager.

Dress warmly. Use long underwear even in the spring and autumn.

Place a space heater or heat lamp in your bathroom and turn it on before showering in the morning.

Stand by the radiator to warm up, or build a fire in the fireplace.

COMFORT

When sitting for long periods of time is necessary, such as when flying, you can relax your back muscles by doing the following. Place your forearms on your thighs, hands near the knees, and lean forward with your face as near to the knees as possible. Breathe deeply and relax in this position. Repeat several times.

Purchase a padded toilet seat, or sew a cover for it out of thick, furry material.

Pad chairs with pillows or foam cushions.

If you don't want to take a pillow with you when going out, take a sweater or jacket along to use as a cushion for hard chairs.

Pain at the base of the toes may be alleviated by placing a bar behind the ball of the foot on the shoe sole. This will allow you to avoid the painful area by rolling off the bar. You should talk to your doctor, chiropodist, or physiotherapist about this before experimenting. It is called a *metatarsal bar*.

Painful feet may also benefit from orthopaedic inserts. Ask your doctor or chiropodist about them.

Recliner chairs with head supports are comfortable for many people, especially if you have neck problems.

Electric beds are no longer confined to the hospital. Home models are available that have movable back and foot sections.

Be sure that you have adequate lighting and ventilation for all activities.

If you take aspirin for pain, you may want to wake up earlier than necessary, take your aspirin, and go back to sleep until it begins to work. Keep aspirin and a glass of water at the bedside.

Splints, often made for hands and from special plastics, help to maintain proper joint alignment, prevent stress, and reduce pain. Your doctor can refer you to an occupational therapist who can construct one for you.

A crêpe bandage can also provide some added stability to joints, as well as serve as a reminder to protect them.

MISCELLANEOUS

To control lamps, equipment, and appliances in inaccessible locations, there is a plug on the market with an on-off switch. This can plug in directly to a wall outlet or can be attached to an extension cord that can be positioned near you.

For those patients whose mobility is very severely limited a Home Control Unit or Possum (from POSM—Patient Operated Selector Mechanism and possum = I can in Latin) is available. This consists of a command console with a number of module units for each appliance wanted. Pushing the buttons on the console will turn any appliance on or off anywhere in your house. These units are expensive but may enable the severely disabled to lead an independent life and thus cover their cost quite quickly.

Use a clipboard to keep writing paper steady.

A felt-tip pen allows you to write with less pressure.

Reachers extend your reach from two to three feet, allowing you to retrieve from the floor or on high shelves.

When attending lectures, use a cassette recorder to eliminate note taking.

When shaking hands with another person, grasp the fingers of the person's hands first so that his or her thumb cannot grasp and squeeze your hand too hard.

Use a steak or paring knife at dinner since the sharper the knife, the less pressure needed. Be careful.

Make sure that the chairs you use at home are easy to get out of—if not, you may not want to get out of them often enough to move around and loosen up. Avoid soft, low chairs.

Dialing a phone may be easier with a
pencil held in the palm of the hand.
Push-button dialling phones are
easier to use and readily available.

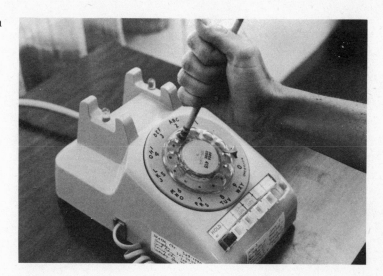

Enlarged knobs are available to
place on lamps as well as appliances
such as washing machines (certain
brands only) to increase ease of
handling. Check with your
washing-machine manufacturer if
the controls are difficult to
operate.

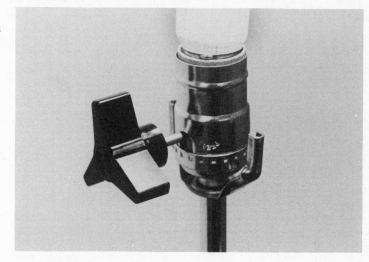

8

Relaxation Techniques

So much has been said and written about relaxation that most of us are completely confused. It is not a cure-all, but neither is it a hoax. Rather, like most treatment methods, it has specific uses in the management of arthritis. The advantage of relaxation is that your muscles become less tense and thus it is easier and less painful to move the joints. In addition to the release of residual tension throughout the body, these techniques are useful in helping you sleep. Relaxation exercises seem to be particularly helpful in relieving pain.

Like exercise, the following techniques take practice. Thus, if you do not feel you are accomplishing anything, be patient and keep trying. Feel free to try another method if the one you have chosen does not seem to work for you, but give it a full week trial. Relaxation techniques can be practiced at any time of the day. With many forms of arthritis, it is wise to take short rest periods during the day to avoid undue fatigue and to relieve stress on the joints. This is an excellent time to practice relaxation techniques.

The following are examples of relaxation techniques. Once you choose the one that works best for you, it may be helpful to tape record the technique. This is not necessary but is sometimes helpful if you find it hard to concentrate or follow the routine. With an inexpensive cassette recorder, you can make a tape to follow so that you don't have to think hard or look at this book while you are trying to relax.

JACOBSON PROGRESSIVE RELAXATION

Many years ago, a psychiatrist, Edmund Jacobson, discovered that if a person wants to relax he or she must learn what it feels like to be relaxed and to be tense. Thus, he designed a very simple set of exercises to assist with the learning process. Jacobson felt that if one could recognize tension he or she could then let it go and relax. Progressive relaxation is best done lying on your back either on a rug or in bed. However, it can be done seated in a comfortable chair. Choose a quiet time and place where you will not be disturbed for at least fifteen minutes.

Technique for Progressive Relaxation of Each Muscle Group

First, for each muscle group of the arms and shoulders:

- Tense (contract) the muscles, holding until the tension is located (two to five seconds).

- Feel the tension, notice it carefully.

   Now release, let the tension slide away, all away.

- Feel the difference.

- Notice the pleasant warmth of relaxation.

- Repeat this sequence with the same group, but use only about half the tension.

- Repeat again with the same muscle group, but allow little movement so that only slight tension can be detected.

For the muscle groups of the lower limbs, trunk, and face it is only necessary to tense the muscles once, very slightly—just enough to recognize the tension. Then let it slide away. Feel the difference. Notice the pleasant warmth of relaxation.

MUSCLE GROUPS	TENSION EXERCISES
1. Dominant hand	Lift hand and make a fist; relax.
Other hand	Lift hand and make a fist; relax.

2. Dominant arm   Lift arm at shoulder; relax.
   Other arm   Lift arm at shoulder; relax.

3. Shoulders   Shrug shoulders; relax.

Repeat each of the above three times with progressively less tension.

4. Right foot   Bend toes, relax; lift toes, relax.
   Left foot   Bend toes, relax; lift toes, relax.

5. Right leg   Start to bend knee (drag heel up slightly); relax.

   Left leg   Start to bend knee (drag heel up slightly); relax.

6. Buttocks   Squeeze together; relax.

7. Abdomen   Make abdomen tight and hard; relax.

8. Chest and neck   Squeeze shoulder blades together and slightly arch back, pressing head backward; relax.

9. Breathing   Take a slow deep breath and relax completely as you exhale. Repeat two or three times.

10. Upper face and scalp   Raise eyebrows; relax. Close eyes tightly; relax.

11. Centre face   Scowl and wrinkle nose; relax. Widen cheeks and brow; relax.

12. Lower face   Purse lips; relax. Smile; relax. Drop jaw; relax.

13. Breathing   Take a slow deep breath and relax completely as you exhale. Repeat two or three times.

Technique for Progressive Relaxation of the Whole Body*

■   Tense all the muscles together and hold for five seconds.

■   Feel the tension, notice it carefully, then release. Let all the tension slide away.

---

*   Much of this section has been adapted from Gordon Paul, *Insight vs. Desensitization, An Experiment in Anxiety Reduction* (Stanford, Calif.: Stanford University Press, 1966).

- Notice any remaining tension. Release it.

- Take a deep breath. Say "relax" softly to yourself as you breathe out slowly.

- Remain totally relaxed.

- Repeat breathing in and out slowly, saying "relax," staying perfectly relaxed.

- Do this three times.

- The exercise has ended—enjoy the relaxation.

Jacobson emphasizes that the only purpose of voluntarily tensing the muscles is to learn to recognize and locate the tension in your body. Hopefully, you will then become aware of the minor states of involuntary tension and use the same procedure of letting go. Once learned it is unnecessary to tense voluntarily, just locate the tension and let it go.

For people with very painful joints, the Jacobson technique may not be the best exercise for relaxation. If it causes any pain, the pain may distract from the relaxation. If this is the case for you, try the following techniques.

THE RELAXATION RESPONSE

During the early 1970s, Dr. Herbert Benson did extensive work on what he calls the relaxation response. He says that our bodies have several natural states. For example, if you meet a lion on the street, you will probably become quite tense. In fact, the response will be a "fight or flight" response. After extreme tension, the body's natural response is to relax. This is what happens after a sexual climax. As life has become more and more complex, our bodies tend to stay in a constant state of tension. Thus, to elicit the relaxation response, many people need to consciously practice the following exercise.

Four Basic Elements

1. **A quiet environment.** "Turn off" not only internal stimuli but also distractions.

2. **An object to dwell upon or a mental device,** for example, repeating a word or sound like the word *one*, gazing at a symbol like a flower, or concentrating on a feeling, such as peace.

3. **A passive attitude.** This is the most essential factor. It is an emptying of all thoughts and distractions from your mind. Thoughts, imagery, and

feeling may drift into awareness—don't concentrate on them, but allow them to pass on.

4. **A comfortable position.** You should be comfortable enough to remain in the same position for 20 minutes.

Technique for Eliciting the Relaxation Response

1. Sit quietly in a comfortable position.

2. Close your eyes.

3. Deeply relax all your muscles, beginning at your feet and progressing up to your face. Keep them relaxed.

4. Breathe in through your nose. Become aware of your breathing. As you breathe out through your mouth, say the word *one* silently to yourself. Try to empty all thoughts from your mind, concentrate on *one*.

5. Continue for 10 to 20 minutes—you may open your eyes to check the time, but do not use an alarm. When you finish, sit quietly for several minutes, at first with your eyes closed. Do not stand up for a few minutes.

6. Do not worry about whether you are successful in achieving a deep level of relaxation. Maintain a passive attitude and permit relaxation to occur at its own pace. When distracting thoughts occur, try to ignore them by not dwelling upon them, and return to repeating *one*.

7. Practice once or twice daily, but ideally not within two hours after any meal, since digestive processes seem to interfere with elicitation of relaxation responses.

You may have noticed that this exercise is very much like meditation. In fact, meditation has provided the principles of the relaxation response. There is no need to spend a lot of money to learn to meditate. You now know all the steps.

SELF-MASSAGE

Self-massage can be considered a relaxation technique and an aid in managing arthritis. Its benefits include the release of tension, the preparation of the body for exercise by relaxing muscles and joints, and the increase of the circulation of blood throughout the body. Furthermore, proper self-massaging can provide comforting heat and warmth to an affected joint.

Self-massage is a simple procedure and can be performed well with little preparation or practice. For instance, no equipment is necessary; a comfortable position is all you need, so as to reach the desired area of massage. Therefore, you can do self-massage at home, at your place of work, or even while waiting at a traffic light. Massage or baby oil can help your hands to move smoothly over the skin, but oil is not at all necessary. Also, self-massage can be done effectively without even removing your clothes.

The techniques of self-massage include: (1) kneading, as if you were preparing dough to bake in the oven; (2) deep pressure in firm circular motions; and (3) firm pressure with fingertips pressing deeply into the muscles. You can combine these techniques to gain the desired relaxation in your joints.

Now, all you need to do is explore and experiment to find the area of tension and the proper technique for release and relaxation. Try self-massage on your neck, back, shoulders, legs, feet, and fingers.

For information on techniques for specific areas or for massage with a partner, you may want to refer to *The Massage Book*, by George Downing (Harmondsworth. Penguin Books, 1974).

These and other varieties of relaxation (such as hypnosis, self-hypnosis, biofeedback, and autogenic training) are not "scientifically proven" treatments for arthritis, and we make no special claims for them. Many individuals in our classes report substantial benefit from these practices, however, and we feel that they have merit for some if used as an adjunct to and not a substitute for a basic sound program.

A word of caution: Various relaxation techniques are often sold in expensive packages as a cure-all for almost everything. Such expensive courses are not necessary. If you want to take a relaxation course, check the following points to avoid unnecessary expense and disappointment.

1. Is the course offered by a reputable institution?

2. Is the cost reasonable?

3. Are claims or promises made for a cure? If so, look elsewhere.

9
Getting a Good Night's Sleep

Sleep is vital for a healthy outlook toward life and important in caring for ourselves. A comfortable bed that allows ease of movement is the first requirement for a good night's sleep. This usually means a firm mattress of good quality that does not allow the body to sag in the middle of the bed. A bedboard, made of 3/8-1/2 inch plywood, can be placed between the mattress and the box spring to increase firmness. Bedboards can be bought commercially or constructed at home.

A heated waterbed is helpful for some people with arthritis because it supports weight evenly by conforming to the body's shape and because it distributes heat to the joints and muscles. Others find waterbeds uncomfortable, even to the point of generating seasickness. If you are interested, try one out at a friend's home or a hotel for a few nights to decide if it is right for you.

An electric blanket, used at a low heat, is another effective way of providing heat while sleeping, especially for cool or damp nights. If you decide to use one, be sure to read and follow the instructions carefully.

Pillows can be used to increase comfort and provide support. For maximum neck comfort, a small pillow should support the curvature of the neck. A pillow can be placed under the shoulder or, if you are lying on your side, under the upper arm to reduce stress on the shoulder joint. For low back problems, a pillow can be placed under the knees, though this position should not be used continuously for a lengthy period of time. Do not place a pillow under your knees or ankles if you have a knee or hip problem.

Positions that are not recommended if you have a disc problem are lying flat on your back or sleeping face down. A recommended position is the side-lying position, in which you lie on your side with knees bent. In this position it can be helpful to place a pillow between the knees to alleviate stress on the hips and low back. A pillow can also be placed under the upper arm to reduce stress on the shoulder joint. But in most cases your body will tell you the best position. There is no single right way.

If you have ankylosing spondylitis, there are some specific sleep positions that will help prevent deformity and loss of mobility of the spine. Sleep on your stomach or flat on your back. Avoid using high pillows under your head; sleep without a pillow if possible. Place a small pillow between your shoulder blades when you sleep on your back.

Sedatives and sleeping pills should be used with great caution. They are often habit forming, they suppress important stages of sleep, and they may cause depression. They only rarely solve sleep problems; the medication that is taken to control sleep actually may produce a disturbed night's sleep. When you stop them, do so gradually. This is also true of alcohol, which some people use as a sleeping medication.

Anti-inflammatory drugs should be taken as prescribed, with the proper dose taken at bedtime. Painkillers are less desirable and should be used with caution because they do not cure the arthritis but only temporarily suppress the symptoms.

Insomnia is a problem that affects all of us at one time or another. However, it can be a cause of concern if it occurs frequently and involves recurrent daytime fatigue or depression. The causes of insomnia are many, some of which are feelings of anxiety or worry, pain or discomfort due to a medical condition, or an unfamiliar sleeping environment. Other contributing factors may be improper self-treatment or failure to follow the practitioner's recommended dosage or directions for medications. If your sleeping problem continues, you may want to seek a doctor's advice. One note: Older persons need less sleep, so be sure your insomnia is not due to sleeping too much. There is more worry about sleeping problems than there are problems.

Some hints for a more comfortable night's sleep include:

■ Maintain a regular sleep schedule so that you go to bed and awaken at about the same time each night and morning.

■ Use some of the relaxation techniques described in this book or create one of your own that is particularly relaxing to you and will settle the day's thoughts and ease the body's tensions.

■ Wait until you are sleepy and your body is ready and eager to go to sleep; going to bed early to ensure a good night's sleep is often counter-productive.

■ Avoid caffeine (coffee, tea, soft drinks, chocolate) for several hours before bedtime because it can act as a stimulant.

■ Moderate your alcohol intake; alcohol may cause an erratic night's sleep and restlessness.

■ Provide yourself with a comfortable environment. Your environment includes mattress, lighting, noise level, temperature, and ventilation.

■ Try taking a warm bath before going to bed.

If you do wake up with stiffness, try some of the easier exercises of Chapter 5 (or small movements in the pain-free range) right in the bed to reduce discomfort and pain, allowing for a more undisturbed and restful sleep.

10
Depression and Other Problems

Depression is like waking up under a big dark cloud every day. Just when you think that you have it licked, back comes the depression, greater than ever.

One of the most frequent problems associated with arthritis is depression. Depression and pain and concerns about growing old are often part of a vicious cycle. The more depressed you are, the more pain you feel; the more pain you feel, the more depressed you become.

We have already discussed a number of ways to deal with pain, including heat, relaxation, exercise, and medications. It is when you are the most depressed that you need to pay the most attention to these techniques. Continue to do these things when you are feeling well in order to maintain your good spirits. Take your medicine and do your exercises—even if you don't feel like it. But you also want to conquer the depression that is making everything worse.

It is not hard to tell when you have pain. But it is not as easy to recognize when you are depressed. Just as there are many degrees of pain, so there are many different degrees of depression. If your arthritis is a significant problem, you almost certainly have or have had some problems with depression; such problems are normal. Depression is felt by everyone at some time. It is how you handle it that makes the difference. The following 14 signs have to do with depression, and you probably have had some of them, in either mild or severe form. Learn them, because they are not the disease but the reaction to the disease, and you need to be able to cope with them.

1. Loss of interest in friends of activities. Not "being home" to friends, perhaps not even answering the doorbell.

2. Isolation. Not wanting to talk to anyone, only watching television, avoiding friends that you happen to meet on the street.

3. Difficulty sleeping, changed sleeping patterns, interrupted sleep, or sleeping more than usual. Often, going to sleep easily, but awakening and being unable to return to sleep. (It is important to remember that older people need less sleep.)

4. Loss of interest in food.

5. Loss of interest in personal care and grooming.

6. Unintentional weight change, either gain or loss, or more than ten pounds in a short period of time.

7. A general feeling of unhappiness lasting longer than six weeks.

8. Loss of interest in being held or in more intimate sex. These problems can sometimes be due to medications and they are very important, so be sure to talk them over with your doctor.

9. Suicidal thoughts. If your unhappiness has caused you to think seriously about killing yourself, get some help from your doctor, good friends, a minister or priest, a psychologist, or a social worker. These are not things to kill yourself over, and these feelings will pass and you will feel better. So get help and don't let a tragedy happen.

10. Frequent accidents. Watch for a pattern of increased carelessness, accidents while walking or driving, dropping things, and so forth.

11. Low self-image. A feeling of worthlessness, a negative image of your body, wondering if it is all worth it. This too will pass.

12. Frequent arguments. A tendency to blow up easily over minor matters, over things that never bothered you before.

13. Loss of energy. Feeling tired all of the time.

14. Inability to make decisions. Feeling confused and unable to concentrate.

If some of these seem familiar, you may well be depressed. There are at least 11 things that you can do to change the situation. But, being depressed, you may not feel like making the effort. Force yourself or get someone to help you into action. Find someone to talk with. Here are the 11 actions:

1. If you feel like hurting yourself or someone else call your doctor, the Samaritans, a friend, a priest or clergyman or the Social Services. Do not delay. Do it now. These feelings do not mean that you are crazy. Most of us feel this way at one time or another. Often, just talking with an understanding person or health professional will be enough to help you through this mood.

2. Are you taking tranquillizers? These include drugs such as Valium, Librium, reserpine, codeine, sleeping medications, and other "downers." These drugs intensify depression, and the sooner you can stop taking them, the better you will be. Your depression may well be a drug side effect. If you are not sure what you are taking or what the side effects might be, check with your doctor or chemist. Before discontinuing a prescription medication, always check, at least by phone, with the prescribing doctor, as there may be important reasons for continuing its use or there may be withdrawal reactions.

3. Are you drinking alcohol in order to feel better? Alcohol is also a downer. There is virtually no way to escape depression unless you unload your brain from these negative influences. For most people, one or two drinks in the evening is not a problem, but if your mind is not totally free of alcohol during most of the day you are having trouble from this drug.

4. Continue your daily activities. Get dressed every day, make your bed, get out of the house, go shopping, walk your dog. Plan and cook meals. Force yourself to do these things even if you don't feel like it.

5. Go and see friends. Call them on the phone, plan to go to the movies or on other outings. Do it.

6. Join a group. Get involved in a church group, a discussion group at a YWCA or YMCA, a senior citizen club, a community college class, a self-help class, or a senior nutrition program.

7. Make plans and carry them out. Look to the future. Plant some young trees. Look forward to your grandchildren's graduation from college even if they are in kindergarten.

8. Don't move to a new setting without first visiting for a few weeks. Moving can be a sign of withdrawal, and depression often intensifies when you are in a location away from friends and acquaintances. Your troubles may move, too.

9. Take a holiday with relatives or friends. Holidays can be as simple as a few days in a nearby city or a resort just a few miles down the road. Rather than go alone, look into trips sponsored by an Adult Education group, your church, the W.I. or a special interest group.

10. Do 10 to 15 minutes of physical exercise every day.

11. Make a list of self-rewards. Take care of yourself. You can reward yourself by reading at a set time, seeing a special play, or by anything big or small that you can look forward to.

Depression feeds on depression, so break the cycle. The success of everything else in this book depends on it. Depression is not permanent, but you can hasten its disappearance. Focus on your pride, your friends, your future goals, your positive surroundings. How you respond to depression is a self-fulfilling prophecy. When you believe that things will get better, they will.

COMMON PROBLEMS: PAIN, FEAR, FATIGUE, AND SEX

Pain

A survey at the Stanford Arthritis Center asked people about their concerns with arthritis. Not surprisingly, the number one concern is pain. Too often the response to this concern is "learn to live with it." This is easy to say, but hard to do. Thankfully, with a little understanding many things can be done about pain.

Pain in arthritis comes in two ways. First, the active inflammation of the disease can cause pain; most pain in rheumatoid arthritis is of this type. Second, the damaged joints can cause pain even though there is no acute inflammation; this is the kind of pain typically found in osteoarthritis. Of course you can have both kinds of pain at the same time, but usually one or the other will be the most severe.

Active pain from inflammation is best treated by reducing the inflammation, by stopping the active disease process. The anti-inflammatory drugs act on the disease process. Thus, the regular use of prescribed medication is essential to keep the pain in check. Occasionally, for very severe pain an analgesic or painkiller is needed for a short time; the painkiller might include codeine. However, while a painkiller may bring temporary relief, over a period of time it may result in addiction or may cover up the symptoms while the damage to the joint goes on.

Pain from damaged joints will usually not be helped much by medication; therefore it is important to learn nonmedical means of pain management. The following principles are important, and apply to both kinds of pain.

1. We can't do two things at once. Our minds are such that we can't concentrate well on two things at the same time. Thus when you have pain it is important to keep active. Get dressed in your favourite clothes; women put on makeup, men shave. Now do something. Go to work, go out shopping, go to a movie you have wanted to see. All of these activities will make you look and feel good, and will help keep your mind off the pain. If you instead stay at home in your old dressing gown and stay in bed or mope around the house you will have too much time to think about your pain and it will seem worse than it is.

2. Do your exercises. Unless you are in a "flare" and have "hot" joints, your exercises will help. Some of the pain of arthritis is due to stiff, unused muscles. Therefore it is very important to keep your muscles in strong, supple condition. Muscle strength will also help keep your joints stable.

3. Practice relaxation exercises. Relaxed muscles and nerve endings send out fewer pain messages and thus you have less pain.

4. Don't be a martyr. Pain is individual, and it cannot be seen. Therefore, don't be afraid to tell friends and family members that you are in pain. Ask for help in carrying groceries, making beds, or mowing the lawn. Don't worry if people look at you strangely. Remember that people usually can't see your arthritis or tell that it is hurting you. A direct request for help is not being dependent, it is a direct, honest, and often necessary communication.

5. Pain is closely related to stress and depression. Thus, reducing stress and depression will also reduce pain. Sometimes people are not aware of how closely attitude and pain are related. Thus, we suggest a simple exercise. For a week, keep a pain/mood diary like the one on the next page. Each day make a mark to reflect your general pain level and mood for that day. At the end of the week, connect all the pain marks and then all the mood marks. We think that you will be able to see a close connection.

Fear

People with arthritis, especially in early stages, have many fears, particularly the fear of disability or of deformity. First, you should know that most people with arthritis never have any disability or deformity. And even if you do have a mild deformity, it will very seldom be noticed by others. We see what we expect to see, and seldom notice any but the most extreme deformities. To prove this for yourself spend a day carefully observing others for deformity or disability. You will be surprised at how many you find; it is just that usually we don't notice.

PAIN/MOOD DIARY

PAIN

	SUN.	MON.	TUES.	WED.	THURS.	FRI.	SAT.
No Pain							
— — —	— —	— —	— —	— —	— —	— —	— —
Terrible							

MOOD

	SUN.	MON.	TUES.	WED.	THURS.	FRI.	SAT.
Feeling Great							
— — —	— —	— —	— —	— —	— —	— —	— —
Feeling Awful							

Second, don't keep your fear to yourself. Fear feeds on fear and grows into depression. Talk to someone, perhaps a friend, your doctor, or a family member. Often, talking with someone is the best thing that you can do. If you don't feel comfortable talking with any of these people, you may want to call a counselling agency. Seeking help with your fears is a very healthy thing to do; the reality is never as bad as you are afraid it will be.

Fatigue

There is no question about it, arthritis can be very draining of energy. This is particularly true of rheumatoid arthritis, but it can be a problem in any type of arthritis. Thus, know that fatigue is a part of the overall problem and that you are not just imagining it. Know also that fatigue can be a sign of depression, so you should consider whether the fatigue might be lessened by treating the depression.

If the fatigue is caused by your disease then there are several things that you can do.

1. Conserve your energy (see Chapter 6 on joint protection).

2. Do the obvious—rest! Take a short nap once or twice a day. If this is impossible then just relax. Try doing a relaxation exercise.

3. Fatigue, like pain and fear, cannot be seen and is not understood by most people. Therefore tell your boss, friends, and family that fatigue is one of the problems of your arthritis and that you may have to take short rests from time to time. Gain their support in allowing you to rest. Most employers are more than willing to allow a little extra rest time for good employees. You, your family, your friends, and your employer should understand that there is a difference between fatigue and being lazy.

4. Take a good long look at yourself. Will you allow yourself to rest? Many of us build our self-images around the false ideal of being indestructible— supermom, macho man, or the perfect worker. If this is you, then reassess your position. Fatigue is one of the body's major early warning systems; it is telling you to take heed. Tune into your own body and follow its directions. The ability to rest is a strength and not a weakness.

Sex

Yes, people with arthritis, even in their seventies and eighties, actively participate in sexual activities. Somehow, when one has a disease the rest of the world thinks that they could not possibly be interested in sex, but this is not true. However, it is true that you may have to be more creative, imaginative, and flexible than most folks, and your partner may have to be more understanding. First, talk over your problems with your partner. No one wants to cause you pain, and by explaining what hurts and what doesn't you can go a long way toward more comfortable sex. Good sex includes good communication so be sure your communications are up to date. Second, try several positions until you find those most comfortable for you. Also, you may want to try other ways than intercourse of expressing sexuality. Finally, remember that there are no hard and fast rules. Beware of simplistic advice — these solutions are usually highly individual. For more information and for illustrations see some of the books listed in the Bibliography.

One final word: Sex can actually help the pain of arthritis. It seems that the excitement of sex stimulates our bodies to produce cortisone, adrenalin, and other chemicals that help to ease pain naturally; use this information as you see fit!

A note about partners of people with arthritis. Many husbands and wives have told us how hard it is to watch their spouse suffer with arthritis. They feel helpless and sometimes guilty that they can't in some way share in their partner's distress. It is hard to live with arthritis, even if you don't have it. We suggest that you talk these problems over with other partners of people with arthritis. You can find such folks through your doctor, arthritis classes, or Arthritis Care. The important thing is to know that you are not alone and that your feelings are normal.

11
What about Those Diets?

The area of foods, diet, and nutrition is one of special concern to many people with arthritis. People have many questions—"Will this food help my arthritis?" "Is there any food I should avoid?" "How can I lose weight?"—and reliable answers aren't always easy to find. In this chapter we will try to answer the basic questions and show how food and nutrition really fit into the picture.

WHAT IS "GOOD NUTRITION," ANYWAY?

To understand what is meant by good nutrition and what it has to do with good health, let us examine what is meant by the words *diet, nutrients,* and *nutrition.* Your diet is simply what you eat and drink each day. Nutrients are the many substances in your food that your body needs to work correctly. When we speak of nutrition, we mean your diet, the nutrients in it, and the whole process whereby the nutrients are used by your body. Good nutrition, then, means giving your body all the nutrients it needs, in the right amounts (not too much, not too little), when it needs them.

125

HOW CAN GOOD NUTRITION HELP ME?

Good nutrition helps everyone. It can help you feel fit and energetic rather than tired and weak. If you have special problems with weight or with water retention, it can help solve them. In general, good eating habits can help you feel and be as healthy and full of life as possible.

If you have arthritis, can a good diet be especially helpful? The answer is both yes and no. No special foods or diets will cure your arthritis or make it go away. However, by helping you deal with other problems (such as over-weight) and helping you feel more fit, proper nutrition can help you cope better with arthritis.

WHAT NUTRIENTS DOES MY BODY NEED?
WHY DO I NEED THEM?

Your body needs many nutrients (over 40 of them) to stay healthy. It is impractical to list all the nutrients and their uses, but the list below is a rough guide. Remember that the nutrients are spread throughout the foods we eat. No one food is "complete" or perfect, but many contain several nutrients.

BASIC NUTRIENT	PURPOSE
1. Water	Water is the "main ingredient" of your body. Water provides the proper environment for the processes that go on inside your body.
2. Carbohydrates	Carbohydrates are what we usually call sugars and starches. Carbohydrates are a main source of energy (calories). They serve as the main fuel for your body's activities.
3. Proteins	Proteins are needed for growth and for the maintenance and repair of your body's tissues (muscles, organs, bones, etc.). They also supply energy and calories.
4. Fats	Fats serve as a source of energy and as a source for certain vitamins. The fat in your body is a form of stored energy, like a reserve fuel supply.

5. Vitamins	Vitamins help control and regulate the various processes that go on in your body. Each vitamin has certain specific tasks and roles in the body, which do not change. Vitamins do *not* supply energy.
6. Minerals	Minerals help control and regulate certain body activities. They also have a role in building and repairing tissues.
7. Fibre	Fibre helps with the regulation of bowel function.

WHAT'S THE BEST WAY TO GET THE NUTRIENTS I NEED?

Just choose wisely which foods you eat. You might think that this is difficult, since there are so many nutrients. But actually, it isn't hard if you follow these guidelines.

Guideline 1. Think of calories as a "currency," like money. Depending on your size, your age, and your physical activity you have a certain number of calories you can "spend" each day on foods and still maintain a good weight. (Those of us who are fairly inactive probably have from 1500 to 2500 calories to spend each day.) With the calorie "budget" you have, you need to include all the nutrients your body needs.

If your calorie budget is small (as it is when you aren't very active, or are trying to lose weight), you need to shop around for "nutrition bargains"— foods that supply many nutrients, yet have relatively few calories. You simply can't afford to spend calories on "luxury" foods that don't provide many nutrients. If you do want an occasional luxury food, or a little more freedom from bargain hunting, you need to increase the number of calories you have to spend. The best way is to increase your physical activity.

Guideline 2. Think of the variety in your diet as your "good nutrition insurance." It is possible to eat just a few foods and have an adequate diet, but it is difficult. People whose diets are varied have a better chance of getting all the nutrients they need.

The reason variety helps is that no food gives you every nutrient, and many only give you a few. When you eat only a few foods, you may be getting a lot (even too much) of a few nutrients and very little of the rest. If you eat many different foods, you are probably getting moderate amounts of many nutrients, which is better.

Guideline 3. Think about making a few changes in your general eating habits. Most of us would be healthier if we cut down on the salt, fat, and sugar we eat and added more *complex carbohydrates*. Complex carbohydrates include fruits and vegetables, plus what we usually think of as starches (breads, cereals, grains, etc.). One benefit of these foods is that many of them (especially fruits, vegetables, and whole-grain products) provide fibre, which promotes proper bowel function. Refined sugars and sweets are not complex carbohydrates.

Many older adults cut back on fruits and vegetables because they feel that some of these cause constipation. Nothing is further from the truth. It is important to use these liberally in your diet.

Guideline 4. Keep the following Consumer's Guide to Eating in mind when you purchase, prepare, and eat your meals.

Things to Remember when Using the Consumer's Guide to Eating

1. The serving sizes and number are only a basic pattern. If you are quite active, you may need to add more food. If you are very sedentary, you may need to focus on the lower-calorie foods in each group.

2. Variety is important. Don't depend on just one or two foods in each group. Experiment a little.

3. Try not to add much fat or sugar to the foods you eat, especially if you are trying to lose weight.

4. Don't eliminate the milk products. People with arthritis still need calcium, and calcium is hard to get without dairy products.

5. Vegetables and fruits will be more nutritious if they are cooked in only a small amount of water.

6. You don't need to buy expensive foods or "health foods" to be well nourished. There are relatively inexpensive nutritious foods in every group.

7. If you are watching your food costs, it can be helpful to cut down on the number of prepared convenience foods you eat and/or eat less meat and more meat substitutes.

8. Consider using meat substitutes. Many people think that they need to eat meat every day. Actually, what they need is to get enough high-quality protein each day. Protein is composed of smaller units called *amino acids*. There are nine amino acids that your body needs but cannot make. High-quality protein is protein that contains these nine amino acids in the right proportions to meet human needs.

THE CONSUMER'S GUIDE TO EATING FOR GOOD NUTRITION

Food Group	Includes	Is a Major Source of	Approximate Serving Size	Number of Servings Needed per Day
Grains and cereals	Whole grain or enriched cereals, grains (including rice), breads, rolls, pasta, etc. (not cakes, biscuits, pastries, etc.)	Carbohydrate, fibre, B vitamins	1 slice bread, or ½ cup cooked cereal or grains, or 1 oz. dry cereal (about ¾-1 cup for many cereals)	4 or more per day
Vegetables and fruits	All vegetables and fruits (pure juices may be used, but should not entirely replace whole foods) (avocados and olives are high in fat, high in calories)	Carbohydrate, fibre, iron, vitamin A, vitamin C	½ cup or 1 medium-size piece of fruit *Vitamin C* rich foods: citrus fruits, canteloupe, tomatoes, strawberries, raw cabbage, potatoes, leafy green vegetables *Vitamin A* rich foods: dark green vegetables (broccoli, kale, chard, spinach, etc.), deep yellow or orange fruits and vegetables (pumpkin, carrots, squash, apricots, sweet potatoes, etc.)	4 or more per day, including: 1 vitamin C food per day; 1 vitamin A food several times a week
Milk products	Milk (low-fat or skim preferred), cheeses (including cottage cheese), yogurt (plain has less sugar), ice cream (for occasional use) (not butter, cream, cream cheese; these are high in fat, relatively low in other nutrients)	Protein, calcium and phosphorus (minerals), riboflavin (a vitamin)	1 cup milk or yogurt, or 1-1½ oz. cheese, or 1/3 cup nonfat dry milk powder, or 1-1½ cups cottage cheese	2 or more per day
Meats and meat substitutes	Meat (preferably lean, trimmed of fat), poultry, fish, eggs, nuts (including peanut butter), legumes (dried beans and peas)	Protein, iron, B vitamins	3 oz. (excluding the bone) of cooked meat, fish, or poultry, or 2 eggs, or 4 tablespoons of peanut butter, or 1 cup dried beans or other meat substitute prepared appropriately	2 or more per day
Other foods	Fats, oils, sugar, sweets, alcohol	These foods supply few nutrients	Limit the amount eaten	You probably get more than enough without adding anything

Meat, milk, and eggs all provide high-quality protein. Most vegetables and grains don't provide high-quality protein when eaten by themselves. This is because the proportions of amino acids in plant proteins often don't match the proportions that people need. However, if several plant foods are combined properly in a meal, the body can get high-quality protein, because one food's amino acids "fill in the gaps" the other leaves.

Legumes and grains are a good example of two vegetable products that "match" or complement each other very well. Legumes (dried beans and peas) are relatively low in two amino acids that grains have plenty of, and grains are low in two amino acids that legumes can provide.

The following ten combinations of plant products will provide good, usable protein.

beans and rice	rice, soybeans, and wheat
beans and corn	peanuts, wheat, and milk
beans and wheat	peanuts, soybeans, and sesame
beans and sesame	peanuts and sunflower seeds
rice and sesame	greens and converted rice (look for the word *converted* on the package)

HOW ABOUT VITAMIN AND MINERAL SUPPLEMENTS? ARE THEY A GOOD WAY TO MAKE SURE I GET THE NUTRIENTS I NEED?

Depending on supplements is not a good idea. The five reasons for this are listed below. The same comments usually apply to cereals and other foods that are "fortified" with several vitamins and minerals.

1. Your body needs many nutrients, not just a few. When you take a supplement, you get only a few of the essential nutrients. The rest are ignored.

2. Supplements can give people a false sense of nutritional security. Some people feel that once they take their pill (or pills) they are "okay" for the day. So they don't think about the nutritive value of the foods they eat. They may end up with worse nutrition than they would have had if they hadn't taken the supplement.

3. Supplements tend to be expensive. Most people would be better off spending more on healthy foods, where money buys many nutrients, than on special supplements, where several pounds may buy only a few nutrients.

4. It is possible to get "too much of a good thing." Some vitamins and minerals build up in the body and are hard to get rid of. If people take in too much of these nutrients, health problems can result. Vitamin D is a

good example. Small amounts of the vitamin are necessary to help maintain strength in bones. But too much can cause trouble and even lead to abnormal calcium deposits in the body. Too much vitamin A can also be harmful.

5. We may not know about all the nutrients humans need yet. If you depend on supplements, you get only the nutrients that people, with current knowledge, choose to add. But if you depend on a variety of good foods, you get all the "extras" nature adds. This may be much better.

HOW CAN I USE NUTRITION AND FOODS TO HELP WITH MY ARTHRITIS?

Unless you have gout, there are no specific foods or diets that will cure or directly treat your arthritis. However, there are several things that can help you. Controlling your weight and coordinating your meals with your medications can be helpful. If so advised by your doctor, restricting your salt intake may be useful. Finally, you can help yourself by learning how to critically judge "diet cures" for arthritis, so that you don't fall into any traps.

Controlling Your Weight

If you are overweight, you are putting extra loads and stress on your weight-bearing joints. This makes little sense if you have arthritis—it may make the pain or inflammation worse. Reducing your weight makes more sense—it will ease the strain, lessen the pain, improve your agility, and make you both look and feel better.

Losing weight can be a difficult task, but it is possible. If you need to reduce, perhaps this information will make the job easier.

Calories are essentially a measure of the fuel value of foods. They tell you how much work your body can do with the energy it gets when you eat a particular food. People get overweight and overfat if they eat more calories than their body needs for its activities. To lose weight and fat, they need to consume fewer calories than they use up. If, over a period of time, a person eats 3500 calories less than he or she needs, he or she will lose one pound.

There are no hard and fast rules about how to lose weight successfully, but following these steps may be helpful.

Step 1: Decide to lose weight and to change your eating habits. People are rarely successful in achieving permanent weight loss if they lack strong commitment to the idea. Check with your doctor to make sure that he or she recommends that you lose weight.

Step 2:   Before you start, think about why you are overweight. Doing this may give you some clues about things you can do to help yourself. For example:

■ Some people eat too much because cooking is one of their hobbies. They enjoy eating a great deal. For them, it may help to prepare less food and to serve smaller portions.

■ Some people are overweight because they (over)eat when they get into a certain mood. They eat when they get depressed, bored, or nervous. In these cases, it may be important for people to find and plan something else to do when the mood strikes.

■ Some people eat large amounts of food almost unconsciously while they do other things. For them it is important to focus on the foods they eat, to eat slowly, and not to do anything else while they eat.

■ Some people are overweight not because they eat so much more than anyone else, but because they aren't as active. In this situation, you should try to increase your physical activity; and you also should accept the fact that you may need to regularly eat much less than others if you want to have a normal, moderate weight.

It may be easier for you to analyze your habits if you write down everything you eat for several days on a record like this:

DAY AND TIME	WHAT I ATE	HOW MUCH I ATE	WHERE I ATE	WHAT MOOD I WAS IN	WHAT I WAS DOING BESIDES EATING

Step 3: Reduce your consumption of the "luxury" foods—high-calorie foods with little nutritive value. In general, these are the foods that are not mentioned as part of the four basic groups in the Consumer's Guide to Eating.

Step 4: Use the basic foods that are lower in fat and sugar content wherever possible. Eat leaner meats, use low-fat or skim milks and cheeses. Avoid fruits canned in heavy syrup.

If necessary, eat smaller portions of the basic foods, but do not eliminate any food group. Many "low-carbohydrate" diets exclude breads and cereals as well as milk and dairy products. Do not use "crash" diets. They deprive your body of many of the nutrients it needs to be healthy, and rarely result in any long-term weight loss.

Step 5: Aim to lose weight gradually. A rate of no more than one or two pounds lost per week is best for most people. (Beware of diets that promise large, quick weight losses. With some of them, including low-carbohydrate diets, you will lose weight rapidly, but much of the loss will be water. The water will be regained quickly after you go off the diet. The aim is to lose fat, not water, so don't be deceived.)

Step 6: Don't be upset if your weight doesn't drop dramatically during the first week or if it reaches a plateau for a few weeks. When you diet, your body doesn't just burn up fat—it goes through many changes. Some of the adjustments it makes may involve changing the amount of water in your body temporarily, and this can affect your weight. But as long as you are eating less than you use up, you will be losing fat. The loss will eventually show up on the scale. If it doesn't, you are still eating too much for you. A further decrease in amount and an increase in discipline are needed.

Some additional comments on losing weight:

1. Eat slowly. When you eat slowly, you give your body time to signal you that you've eaten enough. If you eat rapidly, your body can't respond in time. By the time it tells you to stop, you've probably eaten too much.

2. Try eating small, frequent meals rather than one or two relatively large meals. This tends to help people eat less and feel more satisfied.

3. Special "dietetic" foods are not necessary. They are generally expensive and are not necessarily nutritious.

4. Try to avoid foods that contain a lot of fat or sugar and few nutrients. Sometimes you can recognize these foods because they are greasy, "rich," or very sweet. Some specific examples are:

   - sugar and sweets, cakes and biscuits
   - butter, margarine, cream
   - gravies, sauces, dressing
   - fried foods
   - soft drinks, alcoholic beverages

5. Substitute low-calorie foods for your usual snacks and desserts. Some possibilities:

   - meat or vegetable broths and bouillons
   - vegetable soups (except cream soups)
   - fruits (raw or canned in their own juice)
   - raw vegetables, including unsweetened pickles
   - coffee or tea (plain)

6. Remember that no single food is necessarily "fattening" or "slimming." Since all foods have calories, eating too much of any food can make you gain weight. Moderation in your total intake is the key.

Coordinating Meals and Medications

Many of the drugs used for arthritis have some relationship to food intake and meals. Some of the drugs are best absorbed on an empty stomach. Others may cause stomach problems unless you take them with meals. When you get a new medication, check with your doctor or read Chapter 12 in this book to see whether you should take it with meals. Remember that if your physician asks you to take the drug "with every meal," he or she is probably assuming that you eat three meals a day. If you don't, be sure to tell the doctor so that any necessary adjustments can be made.

Aspirin is one example of a drug that should be taken with meals and with lots of fluids. Doing this helps prevent stomach irritation and upset.

Limiting Your Salt Intake

Salt (sodium chloride) plays many important roles in our bodies. We need sodium for our muscles and nerves to work properly. Sodium can attract and hold water, so we use it to keep the right amount of water in our bodies.

Some people, however, have too much water in their bodies. This can happen when people have high blood pressure. It can also happen when people take certain drugs, including some of those used with arthritis. In such cases, a physician may prescribe a low-sodium diet to help solve the problem.

If you have been asked to limit the amount of sodium in your diet, the following guidelines should be helpful.

1. Reduce the amount of table salt in your food.
   - Reduce the amount of salt used in cooking.
   - Don't use the salt cellar at the table.
   - Remember that many foods already have salt added when you buy them. Read the labels.

2. Remember that other substances besides salt contain sodium.
   - Become a label reader; look for the word *sodium*. *Sodium benzoate*, *sodium bicarbonate* (baking soda), and *monosodium glutamate* are examples of ingredients you may find.

3. The following foods generally contain a great deal of sodium and should be avoided.
   - Processed, cured, smoked, and canned meats
   - Salty popcorn, pretzels, crackers, nuts, potato crisps, and so on
   - Canned soups, bouillon
   - Pickles, sauerkraut, and other foods treated with a brine
   - Some condiments, catsup, and spicy sauces (read the label)

Evaluating Diets and "Cures" for Arthritis— How to Keep from Getting Trapped

We have already mentioned that there are no known nutritional cures for arthritis. No specific foods or nutrients make arthritis better or worse, except in the case of gout. Yet, diet "cures" for arthritis appear regularly in magazines and books, and many people are interested. At the Arthritis Center we have studied the effects of diets; those who follow these fad diets do not feel any better than those who do not.

If you are interested in learning how to read articles and books on "miracle" cures so that you can judge things for yourself and not get "trapped" into unhealthy practices, this final section is for you.

Steps to Follow in Evaluating a Report of a "Cure"

Step 1: Get a copy of the book or article where the originator of the diet explains the diet and the "proof" of its effectiveness.

Step 2: Read the article, focusing on the evidence or "proof." Figure out what kind of evidence the author has. Does he or she try to persuade you with anecdotes—short stories of what happened to individual patients? Or does he or she present the results of scientific studies ("clinical trials")?

Step 3: Evaluate the evidence by asking yourself the following questions.

Questions for Anecdotes (Case Reports)

A. Get the facts.

1. Who was involved?

2. What was the treatment?

3. What was the result? Were there any side effects from the treatment?

4. What claims did the author make, based on this result?

B. Think about the facts, asking yourself:

1. Could anything else have caused the claimed results?

   ■ Was anything besides the diet changed (medications, exercise)?

   ■ Could the change be a result of a psychological effect—"positive thinking" on the part of the patient?

   ■ Could it have been a coincidence? Arthritis pain tends to come and go.

   People often try new cures when they have the most pain, then improve and think the cure works, when it really does nothing. Usually, the improvements actually come about because the arthritis is at the "peak" of the pain cycle when he or she tries the "cure." The arthritis would improve with or without the "cure," simply because the arthritis was going into remission anyway.

2. Were the patients different from other arthritics or from you in any important ways?

3. If the author presents several anecdotes as evidence, are there any patterns, other than that the patient followed the diet and improved? In one currently popular book that deals with nutrition and arthritis, the author presents a number of cases in which patients followed a specific

diet and improved. But if one looks closely, there is another pattern—many of the patients also lost considerable amounts of weight. This sort of thing should make you suspect that maybe it isn't the specific diet but rather the weight loss that caused the improvement.

Questions for Clinical Trials (Studies)

When you read anecdotes, you will probably find that it is difficult to answer the questions suggested above. Observations of single "cases" simply do not give enough information to tell whether treatments really work. That is the reason clinical trials are done—they help us sort out the effects of the treatment from psychological effects, coincidence, and other such things.

A clinical trial is an experiment in which one group of people gets a treatment ("Treatment X"), a similar group gets no treatment or a "traditional" treatment, and the results for the two groups are compared. If the group with the new treatment does better than the other group (the "control" group), the conclusion is that the new treatment helps. But if roughly the same proportion of people get better in both groups, the conclusion is that the new treatment has no effect or at least no more effect than the old treatment.

The following diagram may make the situation clearer. In this case, the conclusion is that Treatment X does not help, because the same number of people got better in both groups. But notice that if the researcher had only looked at the people getting Treatment X (as in case reports), he or she would probably have made the opposite (wrong) conclusion, that the treatment does help.

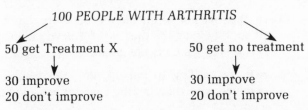

100 PEOPLE WITH ARTHRITIS

50 get Treatment X   50 get no treatment

30 improve   30 improve
20 don't improve   20 don't improve

Here are some questions to ask yourself when people present results from clinical studies.

1. Were the two groups of people really similar? If they were not, the differences between them might have confused the study, making it give deceptive results. For example, if the

group receiving no treatment has more severe arthritis, its members may not improve as much as members of the other group, whose problems are less severe. If this happens, the study may make it seem that Treatment X works better than no treatment, even though it really makes no difference. (Some things that may need to be similar in compared groups are age, sex, weight, exercise and activity patterns, and severity and type of arthritis.)

2. Were the researchers looking for a specific result? If they really wanted to prove that one group did better than the other, it may have biased them, affecting the way they saw things. ("You see what you want to see" can apply to research too, if you're not careful.)

3. Is the study published anywhere in a recent scientific journal? Editors of such magazines usually check and screen articles quite thoroughly. If a study is not published, it may mean that there are real flaws in the procedures used.

Step 4: If you are still not sure whether you should try the diet (after you evaluate the evidence), try to contact your doctor or a dietician to get advice.

Step 5: If you are unable to contact anyone, or if you still think that the diet may be good, ask yourself these questions:

1. Does the diet eliminate any of the basic foods or nutrients? (If so, you may well be harming your health if you follow it.)

2. Does the diet stress only a few foods, so that you will have few calories left to "spend" on the basic foods? (Again, if it does, you may be harming your health.)

3. Do the foods or supplements cost more than you can afford? (If so, following the diet may force you to cut back on other essentials, which is not good.)

4. Are you willing to put up with the trouble and expense involved, knowing that the chances are good that it won't be a cure?

If you answer no to the first three questions and yes to the last, it probably won't harm you to try the diet and see if it works for you. Remember, though, that even if it does seem to work for you, it may not work for someone else.

12

The Drug Scene
KNOW ABOUT THE MEDICATIONS THAT HELP ARTHRITIS

Knowing about your drugs is not easy. No drug is simple and a full explanation from your doctor invariably takes a lot of time. Unfortunately, that time is not always available. The interview with your doctor is an intensive experience. All too frequently discussion of the prescribed treatment serves as a quick end to the encounter. Too little time is spent on this important subject. Here, the discussions you have been having with your physician are repeated. Read the ones you need. Reread those you forget.

DRUGS TO REDUCE INFLAMMATION

The most important arthritis medicines reduce inflammation, and you have to know a little bit about this concept. Inflammation is part of the normal healing process. The body increases blood flow and sends inflammatory cells to repair wounded tissues and to kill bacterial invaders. The inflammation causes the area to be warm, red, tender, and often swollen. To understand the potential problems of drugs that reduce inflammation, it is important to recognize that inflammation is a normal process.

In rheumatoid arthritis the inflammation causes damage and thus suppression of the inflammation can be helpful in treatment. In osteoarthritis there is little inflammation or the inflammation may be necessary for the healing process. So you don't always want an anti-inflammatory drug just because you have arthritis—in rheumatoid arthritis, yes; in osteoarthritis, probably no.

Drugs are known either by their brand name or by their approved name. There is also a much longer chemical name which need not concern us. One drug with a single approved name may be known by a variety of brand names. Doctors are encouraged under the National Health to use the approved name as this allows the chemist to give the cheapest or whichever brand he has in stock. A doctor may wish to stipulate a particular brand on occasions for clinical reasons. The brand names tend to be shorter and more easily remembered than the approved names and are more convenient to use but, as can be imagined, this system causes some confusion to patients unfamiliar with it.

ASPIRIN

The most familiar drug that you will come across in the treatment of arthritis is aspirin. It is also the most useful. It is a member of a group of drugs called salicylates, other members of which are also of great benefit to arthritics. By its very familiarity it does not get the respect it deserves and is sometimes used as a symbol of a doctor's neglect: "Take two aspirin and call me in the morning." It is not without dangers, however, and these are often greatly exaggerated by scare stories in the press. While pretending to act in patients' best interest, these stories are more likely to prevent patients getting the full benefit of a most potent drug, than alert them to hidden dangers. The following day the same press reports that aspirin may prevent heart attacks by thinning the blood. These contradictions dominate our daily encounters with aspirin.

Aspirin has two major beneficial effects: pain killing or analgesic, and anti-inflammatory.

It is in the first role of a pain-killer that aspirin will be most familiar to the majority of the population. Aspirin is one of the most frequently found drugs in the family medicine cabinet, useful for a variety of minor ailments, headaches, toothache and feverish chills. For these purposes one or two tablets (300 mg–600 mg) is the usual dose and the effect will last some four to six hours.

In rheumatoid arthritis, while not neglecting its analgesic properties, we are more interested in its anti-inflammatory action. For this purpose a much larger dose is required, usually 12 to 14 tablets (300 mg each) per day and the process must be continued for three to four weeks to obtain the full effect. In these doses medical supervision is necessary and it is not uncommon to meet with some side effects.

The standard aspirin tablet is 300 mg and is insoluble. If you can tolerate this form of the drug, it is just as beneficial therapeutically as any other and is much the cheapest. Some people prefer to use a soluble form which they can take as a drink in a glass of water. Aspirin can be intensely irritating to the lining of the stomach in susceptible individuals, particularly those with a past history of chronic indigestion or peptic ulcer (a gastric or duodenal ulcer). This can be lessened by the use of enteric-coated aspirin which are not absorbed in the stomach but further down the intestinal tract. This does not always work: either the coating does not dissolve and the tablet is passed right through the system or the coating dissolves too soon so that the uncoated aspirin can still irritate the stomach before it passes on. The aspirin circulating in the blood, no matter where it was absorbed, is enough to irritate the stomach in some patients. Taking an antacid or taking the aspirin after a meal helps to slow down the rate of absorption and minimize the irritant effect on the stomach. If, despite the above advice, you get prolonged stomach pain or blood in the stools, usually evidenced by a loose stool of a black tarry nature (a melaena stool) you should stop taking aspirin immediately and consult your doctor.

Many people confuse allergy and side effects of drugs. Being allergic to a drug means that you are abnormally sensitized to it. Even a very small amount rings the alarm bells in your system which over-reacts, producing such symptoms as a skin rash, a runny nose or a wheeze in the lungs. People with a history of asthma have a leaning towards allergic reactions and must be careful of aspirin which may produce an exacerbation of their symptoms. In another context, as an illustration, hay fever is an allergic reaction to grass pollen.

Side effects are different. When considering the action of a drug we concentrate on its beneficial effects, but no drug is that simple, acting in one way only. There will always be a number of other effects on different organs and systems of the body. These are known as side effects and everyone will experience them if they get enough of the drug. Fortunately allergy to aspirin is rare but if present it is likely to be there with other members of the salicylate group of drugs. Side effects can usually be overcome by reducing the dose or taking the drug in another form.

To get the maximum benefit from aspirin it is often necessary to work the dose up to that which will produce some side effects, the most common being a ringing sensation in the ears, and then reduce it until the unpleasant effects are diminished.

Aspirin produces some blood loss through the bowel in most people due to its prolonging of the blood clotting mechanism. The blood can only be detected by sensitive tests on the stool and should cause no concern, but easily detectable or heavy blood loss should be a cause for contacting your doctor. Drugs are chemicals. Interactions between two drugs (two chemicals) are extremely common. Aspirin blocks absorption from the stomach of some of the newer anti-inflammatory agents discussed later. By and large the fewer medicines you take at one time, the more predictable your response to treatment will be. Most reactions having to do with absorption or interactions with other drugs are not perfectly predictable. You may have them or you may not. The treatment for your arthritis will ultimately be unique to you. You may need to discover by trial and error some of the reactions to your own body.

Remember that although aspirin is a familiar household remedy it is a powerful drug and a potential poison. Overdoses can be hazardous and even a small number of tablets in a young child could be lethal. Be sure to keep your medicines out of the reach of children and preferably in a medicine cabinet with a lock.

OTHER ANTI-INFLAMMATORY DRUGS THAT ARE NOT STEROIDS

Aspirin is a *non-steroidal anti-inflammatory drug* (NSAID). That is, it is not a corticosteroid (like prednisolone) and it is an anti-inflammatory agent because it fights inflammation. But some of the disadvantages of aspirin have been noted above. In anti-inflammatory doses, side effects such as nausea, vomiting and ringing in the ears are common. Some people can't tolerate these side effects. Others, either ill advised or not persistent enough, don't really try. Aspirin requires many tablets and regular attention to the medication schedule. So a class of "aspirin substitutes," given the cumbersome name of non-steroidal anti-inflammatory drugs, has been developed. In common medical usage, aspirin is not included in this group, principally because it was invented before the term was coined. To further simplify, we use the term *anti-inflammatory drugs* in this book. In the over-the-counter market "aspirin substitute" usually refers to paracetamol (Panadol) which is discussed below as a pain reliever; paracetamol is not an aspirin substitute for rheumatoid arthritis.

There is a huge market for drugs of this type. Nearly every drug company has tried to invent one and has promoted heavily whatever has been developed. Many of these drugs are good ones. They may be better for those truly unable to tolerate aspirin. Unfortunately, they are more expensive, newer, and their long-term side effects are less well known. While present evidence suggests that they are slightly safer than aspirin because of fewer stomach problems, they probably should not yet be accepted as less hazardous. Aspirin has been around for a very long time and experience with these newer drugs is sufficiently short for there to be some side effects which may not yet have been discovered.

In perspective, the development of these drugs represents a substantial advance. In part this is because of the difficult problems posed by the corticosteroids (discussed later). The use of the term *non-steroidal* to distinguish these compounds underscores the importance of this feature. In average potency, full doses of these drugs are roughly equivalent to full dose aspirin. Gastric intestinal effects such as heartburn and nausea are usually less frequent than with aspirin—hence an advantage for those with intolerant stomachs. Available evidence indicates that different drugs can be best for different individuals. These drugs come from several different chemical families and are not interchangeable. You may have to try several to find the best. The major medications in this category are discussed below. They are given their approved chemical name with the registered trade mark brand name in brackets.

The salicylate group of drugs all have much the same anti-inflammatory action but differ in their side effects and acceptability. **Aloxiprin (Palaprin forte)** is a form of buffered aspirin and many patients find the tablets, which can be sucked or chewed or swallowed whole, pleasanter to take.
Benorylate (Benoral) consists of the molecules of aspirin and paracetamol joined together in such a way that they do not break apart until after they have been absorbed. This means that there is no free aspirin to irritate while the drug is still in the stomach. It can be taken in either tablet form or as a suspension which is easy to swallow and it is only necessary to take the suspension twice per day.
Trilisate tablets contain **choline magnesium trisalicylate**, a highly soluble non-acetylated salicylate which is more effective than aspirin in reducing pain and inflammation, without the gastro-intestinal side effects usually experienced with aspirin. Trilisate tablets also offer the patient the convenience of a twice-daily dose.

Other members of the salicylate group which may be encountered are **salsalate (Disalcid)** and **sodium salicylate.**

Phenylbutazone used to be one of the most potent anti-inflammatory drugs excluding the salicylates in use in the treatment of rheumatic diseases. It suffers from side effects similar to aspirin noted above, i.e. irritation of the intestinal tract giving rise to nausea and indigestion, but far more seriously, it can cause on rare occasions problems with the blood which can be fatal. The production of the red cells may be interfered with giving rise to "aplastic anaemia," or the white cells may suffer in agranulocytosis.

Fortunately these conditions are very rare and seem to be confined to long courses of the drug, so there is still a place for short sharp courses of phenylbutazone to combat an acute bout of inflammation such as gout.

Oxyphenbutazone is a similar drug.

You may have heard of phenylbutazone as "butes" in connection with racehorses! However, for routine use the newer NSAIDs are preferred to eliminate the toxicity.

Almost as powerful is **indomethacin (Indocid).** It has sufficient potency to cope with the acute inflammation of gout and is also useful in the prolonged inflammation of rheumatoid arthritis. Gastric intestinal irritation can be a problem and some patients complain that indomethacin makes them feel thick-headed or bloated due to fluid retention. The side effects can sometimes be minimized by taking the drug in a slow-release capsule or a suppository as alternatives to the usual 25 mg capsule.

The proprionic acid derivatives are a group of drugs which have been developed since those already mentioned in an effort to avoid the side effects and toxicity. They are usually well tolerated and taken in full dosages are equally effective. The best known are ibuprofen (Brufen), fenoprofen (Fenopron), ketoprofen (Orudis–100 and the new long-acting Oruvail), (Alrheumat), naproxen (Naprosyn).

Other drugs worth mentioning are: (a) the lesser known proprionic acid derivatives; (b) drugs which are related chemically but not strictly to be classified as such; and (c) drugs which fall into no easy classification. They include:

    (a) Flurbiprofen (Froben)
        Fenbufen (Lederfen)

    (b) Fenclofenac (Flenac)
        Diclofenac (Voltarol)
        Diflunisal (Dolobid)
        Sulindac (Clinoril)
        Tolmetin (Tolectin)
        Zomepirac (Zomax)
        Pentazoine (Fortral)
        Mefenamic acid (Ponstan)
        Flufenamic acid (Meralen)

    (c) Piroxicam (Feldene)
        Azapropazone (Rheumox)
        Feprazone (Methrazone)

The list is not exhaustive as new drugs are being added to it continually, and some are withdrawn from time to time either because of failure to catch on commercially or from unacceptable side effects.

They all have their part to play in the treatment of musculo-skeletal disorders. They vary in their length of action—some only have to be taken once or twice a day—and in the incidence of side effects. Gastro-intestinal irritation, and thus caution in the presence of a past history of indigestion or peptic ulcer, skin rashes and exacerbation of asthma are all possibilities, along with ringing in the ears, fuzzy feelings in the head and vertigo.

The last three in the list could equally be listed under the heading of pain killers or analgesics and will be mentioned again.

It is not really possible to say that one drug is better than another; it all depends on the individual response. The positions in the list are purely arbitrary in terms of efficacy; however, the prices of drugs vary enormously and doctors are under an obligation to pay attention to value for money; in this respect humble aspirin wins hands down. Drug companies expend considerable amounts of money in developing new drugs, and when first put on the market have to try to recoup their expenditure. As this phase passes drugs become relatively cheaper and so the older drugs have a benefit in cost and also the added advantage that doctors are more familiar with their use and are better able to predict what side effects are likely to be encountered. So where no very great difference is detectable clinically, doctors should use the least expensive. This is not to say that, when an individual is found to respond clinically much better to one of the more expensive drugs, it will not be given.

CORTICOSTEROIDS

In about 1950, a widely heralded miracle occurred—the introduction of cortisone for the treatment of arthritis. The Nobel prize was awarded to the doctors who developed this drug. Persons with rheumatoid arthritis and other forms of synovitis suddenly noted that the swelling and pain in their joints decreased and that the overall toxicity of the disease disappeared. They felt fine.

The initial enthusiasm for cortisone in arthritis was tremendous. But over the following years, a number of major cautions began to be voiced. Slowly, the cumulative side effects of the cortisonelike drugs began to be recognized. For many individuals, the side effects were clearly greater than any benefits obtained. Cortisone became the model of a drug that provides early benefits but late penalties. Now, with a quarter of a century of experience with these drugs, our perspective is more complete. They represent a major treatment for arthritis, but their use is appropriate in only a relatively small number of cases and then only with full attention to potential complications.

Steroids are natural hormones manufactured by the adrenal glands. When used medically, they are given in doses somewhat higher than the amounts the body generally makes. In these doses they suppress the function of your own adrenal glands and lead to a kind of drug dependency as the gland slowly shrinks. After many months of steroid use, the drug must be withdrawn slowly to allow your own adrenal gland to return to full function, otherwise an "adrenal crisis" can occur in which you just don't have enough hormone. Steroids must be taken exactly as directed and a physician's close advice is always required.

Let's discuss the side effects. They can be divided into categories depending upon the length of time you have been taking the steroid and the dose prescribed. Side effects result from a combination of how high the dose is and how long you have been taking it. If you have been taking steroids for less than one week, side effects are quite rare even if the dose has been high.

If you have been taking high doses for one week to one month, you are at risk for development of ulcers, mental changes including psychosis or depression, infection with bacterial germs, or acne over the skin. The side effects of steroid treatment become most apparent after one month to one year of medium to high dosage. The individual becomes fat in the central parts of the body, with a buffalo hump on the lower neck and wasting of the muscles in the arms and legs. Hair growth increases over the face, skin bruises appear, and stretch marks develop over the abdomen. After years of steroid treatment (even with low doses) there is loss of calcium, resulting in fragile bones. Fractures can occur with only slight injury, particularly in the spine. Cataracts slowly develop and the skin becomes thin and translucent. Some physicians believe that hardening of the arteries occurs more rapidly and that there may be complications of inflammation of the arteries.

Many of these side effects will occur in everyone who takes sufficient doses of cortisone or its relatives for a sufficient period of time. The art of managing arthritis with corticosteroids involves knowing how to minimize these side effects. The physician will work with you to keep the dose as low as possible at all times. If possible, you may be instructed to take the drug only once daily rather than several times daily, since there are fewer side effects when it is taken this way. If you are able to tolerate the drug only every other day, this is even better, for the side effects are then quite minimal. Unfortunately, many people find that the dosage schedules that cause the fewest side effects also give them the least relief.

Steroids are always to be used with great respect and caution. Some experienced doctors still use low-dose corticosteroid treatment in rheumatoid arthritis, demonstrating that the proper indications for use of these drugs are somewhat controversial. High-dose cortisone treatment for uncomplicated rheumatoid arthritis has long been considered bad practice. Corticosteroids are harmful in infectious arthritis and should not be given by mouth in local conditions or in osteoarthritis.

There are three ways to give corticosteroids. They can be taken by mouth, they can be given by injection into the painful area, or an injection of adrenal cortical stimulating hormone (ACTH) can be given to cause an individual's own adrenal gland to increase production of hormones. **Prednisolone** is the steroid usually given by mouth and is the reference steroid discussed here. There are perhaps 20 different steroid drugs now available. Cortisone itself retains too much fluid and the second drug developed, hydrocortisone, has the same deficit. The fluorinated steroids, such as triamcinolone, cause greater problems with muscle wasting than does prednisolone.

Many doctors say that steroids should be used to reduce inflammation on a short-term basis to gain enough time to do something else. Steroids are drugs which must always be used under strict medical supervision. Some of the drugs mentioned up till now, the salicylates and the NSAIDs, could be left to the patient to regulate the dose in accordance with symptoms, but steroids are not like this. Furthermore, because of their effects on other systems of the body, it is imperative that a record is carried by the patient at all times showing that they are on steroids and in what form and dosage in case of emergency treatment. A little card is available which says on the front, "I AM A PATIENT ON STEROID TREATMENT WHICH MUST NOT BE STOPPED ABRUPTLY" to carry in the wallet or handbag and on which doses can be recorded.

Prednisolone, as a little white tablet of either 1 mg or 5 mg, is the most usual method of oral steroid therapy. Also available are brown enteric-coated prednisolone 2·5 mg or 5 mg tablets which are less likely to cause stomach troubles. **Betamethasone** and **dexamethasone** are other steroids which may be used orally.

In addition to giving steroids by mouth, the body can be stimulated to increase the production of its own steroids. This is done by giving adreno-corticotrophic hormone or ACTH.

ACTH (Acthar gel) is given by injection, usually every other day. It produces rapid response in exacerbations of rheumatoid arthritis and can be helpful in some cases as an interim measure whilst awaiting effect from other slower-acting drugs. It is occasionally used for long-term therapy in this disease.

Tetracosactrin (Synacthen depot) is similar in action to ACTH but it is claimed to last longer in the body. However, it may give rise to anaphylactic reactions.

Steroids are sometimes injected into particularly painful joints; however, great care has to be taken to avoid introducing infection into the joint. At the same time fluid may be withdrawn if there has been a build up. The response will give some idea as to how useful this sort of treatment is going to be. If the relief only lasts a few days it is not worth persevering. Injections can only be given at infrequent intervals, say six weeks to three months, as repeated injections can cause local damage and a limit of three injections in a single site is observed by many doctors. Although there are severe limitations to this form of treatment it can be very useful to "unlock" a joint that has become immobile long enough to allow physiotherapy to increase the range of movement, i.e. to reduce inflammation on a short-term basis long enough to do something else as mentioned above.

Hydrocortisone or prednisolone can be used for injection or possibly a longer duration of action is achieved with dexamethasone, methylpredni-solone or triamcinolone.

GOLD SALTS AND PENICILLAMINE

These are major league drugs, although no one knows exactly why they are so effective in so many individuals. Each has major side effects that require stopping treatment for at least one quarter of the users and that may in rare cases be fatal. They are very potent drugs normally prescribed only under the close supervision of a practising consultant rheumatologist who is in a position to carry out the various tests to monitor the effectiveness and possible serious side effects. A general practitioner does not normally originate prescriptions for these drugs.

Gold salts and penicillamine are two very different kinds of drugs, but there are striking similarities in the type and magnitude of good effects and in the type of side effects. Neither appears to be of use in any category other than rheumatoid arthritis, but the scientific proof of their effectiveness in RA is impressive.

These agents can result in remission of the arthritis. In perhaps one quarter of users the disease will actually be so well controlled that neither doctor nor patient can find any evidence of it. Usually these drugs have to be continued in order to maintain the remission, but the effects can be more dramatic than with any other agent to reduce inflammation, except possibly some of the more dangerous immunosuppressant drugs. Individuals who use these drugs must accept certain significant hazards, but there is a good chance of very major benefit. In rheumatoid arthritis, these drugs have been proven to retard the process of joint destruction.

If you are not able to tolerate one of these drugs, you may be able to tolerate the other. If you don't get a good response from one, you may from the other. After failure with one drug, the chances decrease a little, but success with the second drug is still common.

Which should be used first? No one knows. In England, penicillamine is usually used first. In the United States, it is gold. Gold must be given by injection and requires a visit to the doctor every week for a while. An oral form of gold treatment is undergoing trials but is not yet ready for general use.

Penicillamine can be taken by mouth, and while the drug itself is expensive, the total cost may be less. In terms of effectiveness and in risk, you can consider these two drugs about the same.

How Gold is Given
50 mg per week is given by intramuscular injection for 20 weeks, then one to two injections per month thereafter. Many doctors use smaller doses for the first two injections to test for allergic reactions to the injections. Sometimes doctors will give more or less than this standard dosage depending upon your body size and response to treatment. "Maintenance" gold treatment refers to injections after the first 20 weeks (which result in about 1000 mg of total gold). The dosage and duration of maintenance therapy varies quite a bit; with good responses, the gold maintenance may be continued for many years, with injections given every two to six weeks.

Maintenance dosage may be much lower—from 10 to 25 mg. The duration is more important than the dosage.

Side Effects

The gold salts accumulate very slowly in the tissues of the joints and in other parts of the body. Hence, side effects usually occur only after a considerable amount of gold has been received, although allergic reactions can occur even with the initial injection. The major side effects have to do with the skin, the kidneys, and the blood cells. The skin may develop a rash, usually occurring after ten or more injections, with big red spots or blotches, often itchy. If the rash remains a minor problem, the drug may be cautiously continued, but occasionally a very serious rash occurs following gold injections.

The kidneys can be damaged so that protein leaks out of the body through the urine. This is called *nephrosis* or the *nephrotic syndrome* if it is severe. When it is recognized and the drug is stopped, the nephrosis usually goes away, but cases have been reported in which it did not reverse. The blood cell problems are the most dangerous. They can affect either the white blood cells or the platelets, those blood cells that control the clotting of the blood. In each case, the gold causes the bone marrow to stop making the particular blood cell. If the white cells are not made, the body becomes susceptible to serious infections that can be fatal. If the platelets are not made, the body is subject to serious bleeding episodes that can be fatal. These problems almost always reverse when the drug is stopped, but reversal may take a number of weeks, during which time the person is at risk for a major medical problem.

There are other side effects, such as ulcers in the mouth, a mild toxic effect on the liver, or nausea, but they usually are not as troublesome. Overall, about one quarter of users have to stop their course of treatment because of the side effects. One or two per cent of users experience a significant side effect; the other users don't really notice very much of a problem, even though a serious side effect may be about to occur. In less than one in a thousand cases there may be a fatal side effect. With careful monitoring, the drug is reasonably safe and its benefits justify its use, since over 70 percent of those treated with gold show moderate or marked improvement. However, you must maintain your respect for this treatment and keep up regular blood tests to detect early side effects. One final note: most side effects occur during the first initial period of 20 injections. Serious side effects during the maintenance period are unusual.

Special Hints

You must learn to be patient with gold treatment. The gold accumulates slowly in the body and responses are almost never seen in the first 10 weeks of treatment. Improvement begins slowly after that and major improvement is usually evident by the end of 1000 mg or 20 weeks. Similarly, if the drug is stopped, it requires many months before the effect is totally lost. In one famous study, the gold group was still doing better than the control group two years after the drug had been stopped, although most of the effect of the drug had been lost by that time. After a side effect, many doctors will suggest that the drug be tried again. Often, this can be worthwhile if the approach is very cautious, since the drug is frequently tolerated the second time around, although it is not wise to try again if there have been problems with the blood.

To minimize the chance of serious side effects, most doctors recommend that a check be made of the urine for protein leakage, of the white cells and the platelets, and that the patient is questioned about skin rash before every injection. This is good practice.

Penicillamine (Distamine, Cuprimine, Pendramine)
The starting dose is 125 mg or 250 mg daily with increases at monthly intervals up to 500 mg per day, although some patients may need only 250 mg and others up to 1000 mg daily. If a successful remission is achieved, often a lower maintenance dose can be continued indefinitely. If there has been a reaction to gold therapy, penicillamine should be avoided for at least six months.

Side Effects
These closely parallel those noted above for gold injections. The major side effects are skin rash, protein leakage through the urine, or a decrease in production of the blood cells. Additionally, individuals may have nausea, and some notice a metallic taste in their mouth or a decreased sense of taste. Penicillamine weakens the connective tissue so that the healing of a cut is delayed, and a scar may not have the same strength it would have without the penicillamine. So, stitches following a cut should be left in for a longer period of time, and wound healing should be expected to be delayed. Surgery under these circumstances may be more difficult.

Special Hints
Penicillamine takes a number of months to reach its full therapeutic effect and the effect persists for a long time after you stop taking the drug. Responses usually take from three to six months but can be as late as nine months after the drug is begun. Because of the risk of side effects, doctors have now adopted the "go low, go slow" approach given in the dosage schedule above. When full doses were begun earlier, the frequency of side effects was higher. Even now, only about three-quarters of individuals will complete the treatment and the remainder will have some side effects, approximately the same as those listed for gold salts. The drug may be tried again after a side effect if the side effect has been mild. We do not try the drug again if there has been a problem with the blood counts, but may

cautiously try it if there has been a minor problem with protein in the urine, a minor skin rash, or minor nausea.

Monitoring for side effects has to be carefully performed. Usually a blood count or smear, a urinalysis for protein leakage, and questioning of the person about side effects are required every two weeks or even more frequently. It should be noted that with both penicillamine and gold, careful monitoring improves your chances of not having a serious side effect, but does not eliminate them. These drugs contain an intrinsic hazard that no physician can eliminate. Again, after the first six months, side effects are relatively rare but still do occur. Some individuals will have an excellent response to the penicillamine, even though they never get up to the full dosage of 1000 mg per day.

DRUGS TO REDUCE PAIN (ANALGESICS)

There is a selection of drugs to relieve pain which have little or no anti-inflammatory action. At the bottom end of the range are the common analgesics which can be bought at the chemist without a prescription. These are useful as a home remedy for minor aches and pains such as headaches and toothache. At the other end are the powerful morphia derivatives which are highly addictive and whose use has to be strictly controlled by the Misuse of Drugs Regulation 1973. In the middle are drugs to control moderate pain.

Analgesics are relatively little used in rheumatoid arthritis but some physicians use combinations of them with other anti-inflammatory agents. They have more use in osteoarthritis where there is little inflammation to overcome; however, they do have serious limitations. After prolonged use they are found to be less effective and one can get into the situation of requiring increasingly stronger analgesics. Taking strong analgesics can mask pain so that a joint can be injured by over-enthusiastic movement. Most analgesics are constipating which may already be a problem with patients whose mobility has been diminished.

Their best use is to reserve them for short-term problems, particularly when the joint is at rest, so that unintentional injury is avoided.

Paracetamol (Panadol) since its introduction some years back has to a large extent taken over the everyday minor analgesic role of aspirin. Many homes keep paracetamol in stock for day-to-day use. It is similar in pain-relieving power to aspirin but is much less irritant to the stomach. It is available in ordinary tablet form, in a soluble tablet form and as an elixir mainly for use in children. Although usually free from side effects in normal doses (up to 8 tablets in 24 hours), overdosage is particularly dangerous. After an overdose a patient may seem perfectly well for three days only to suffer severe liver damage. Antidotes have now been developed, however, which, if administered within twelve hours, offer every prospect of preventing liver damage. They are availabe to the accident and emergency departments of all major hospitals in the United Kingdom.

Dextropropoxyphene is a useful drug in the middle range for mild to moderate pain. It is usually free from troublesome side effects, although the whole range of stomach problems, skin rashes, dizziness, etc., may occur in some people. The main danger is that the dangerous dose is not very much bigger than the normal therapeutic dose; also, its effect in conjunction with other drugs including alcohol can give rise to concern.

Codeine is a drug which has been around for many years. It is a narcotic drug and can lead to addiction, but because it is a frequent ingredient in many combination drugs this aspect of it is frequently overlooked. It causes constipation readily, to such an extent that it is frequently used as a remedy for diarrhoea.

Dihydrocodeine is a similar drug with a more potent analgesic property than codeine.

The analgesics already mentioned are those most commonly encountered. They are found either singly or in many different combinations with each other, or with aspirin. Again the list is not exhaustive.

Pentazoine (Fortral), mefenemic acid (Ponstan) and **zomepirac (Zomax)** have all been mentioned before. They have an analgesic potency in the middle range, but also have a worthwhile anti-inflammatory action.

Finally, the true narcotic drugs such as Pethidine and Morphia, which are the most potent analgesics, have virtually no place in the treatment of arthritis. They are reserved for acute emergencies.

TRANQUILLIZERS

Diazepam (Valium), chlordiazepoxide (Librium) and other drugs of this nature are some of the most frequently prescribed of all drugs. They do not help arthritis (although diazepam can be used to relieve muscle spasm); they act to depress the patient and they should be avoided by persons with arthritis wherever possible. Any benefit they give to calm the emotions is not sustained.

13
Working with Your Doctor
A JOINT VENTURE

WHICH DOCTOR?

Your main point of contact with the medical profession is likely to be your local family general practitioner. He, in turn, can refer you to a general physician or more specifically, a rheumatologist. A general practitioner, or GP, has special training in taking care of all the common health problems that occur in a family. Thus a GP may assist at the birth of a baby and also take care of grandmother's arthritis.

In choosing a GP, go for the three 'A's: Availability, Affability and Ability.

Whatever degree of disability you have, it is likely to make travelling difficult for you, so do choose a doctor close to where you live. It makes things much easier if the surgery is within easy walking distance, so that your visits to the doctor do not involve the use of public or private transport. There will be times when either or both are not available or are inconvenient. Remember, availability cuts both ways; if you are confined to your house you are much more likely to get frequent visits from your doctor if it does not take a large slice out of his busy day. So if you move house to a neighbouring area, think before putting pressure on your doctor to keep you on his list if it means a long journey for either of you, even though you may have come to like him and know him well.

See if you can get on the list of a GP with whom you can make friends. It is very frustrating being looked after by a brilliant but unapproachable man with whom you are unable to communicate.

Which leaves ability. Obviously you do not want to be looked after by an incompetent doctor, but how do you find out? Well, the letters after his name may be some guide, but unless you know what they stand for, beware, because some of the shortest titles signify some of the highest qualifications, e.g. M.D., and vice versa. Probably the best way to find out is to ask your neighbours. People love to talk about their doctors and you should be able to get a good idea from local recommendations.

A physician is a doctor who has had special postgraduate training in the care of adults. Physicians take care of all the common health problems including arthritis. However, more and more hospitals now have a physician who specializes in arthritis and who is called a rheumatologist. If one is available in your area your GP is likely to choose a rheumatologist if he wishes you to see a consultant.

Since arthritis is a condition frequently seen in general practice, GPs often become expert in handling it and develop it as a special interest, so there may be no need for your GP to seek help from more specialized doctors; however, your GP may want help on specific points and refer you to a specialist for this purpose. When his queries have been answered you can expect to be referred back to your GP, for day-to-day care, although it may be thought wise for you to attend a specialist follow-up clinic for review from time to time. Do not be afraid to ask for a second opinion from a specialist if there are factors you are unhappy about or you think could be improved on. GPs should be and usually are quite happy to seek outside help, as treatment ideally is a co-operative venture.

Your doctor will often enlist the help of two other disciplines within the caring professions, those of the physiotherapist and occupational therapist.

A physiotherapist will help you with exercises, and with means to make movements easier such as heat treatment and massage or hydrotherapy. Physical medicine is at its most effective in dealing with arthritis.

You will find the help of an occupational therapist invaluable in making life easier around the house. For tasks which may seem unsurmountable to you unaided, there are often very simple answers if only you ask the right person, the occupational therapist. Most of the aids already mentioned in this book, and many more, are best obtained through an occupational therapist.

COMMUNICATING WITH YOUR DOCTOR

It is a sad fact that doctors and patients often fail to achieve satisfactory communication. Older doctors seldom had any specific training in making meaningful contact with their patients; it was considered a knack which they either acquired with practice or did not, as the case might be. In recent years it has been realized that communication can be learned, and young doctors are now taught communication as part of their training. Much pioneering work was done by Dr Michael Balint who helped to make doctors aware of their shortcomings, but there is still great room for improvement. Doctors and patients look at a consultation from different sides and they do not always meet in the middle. The doctor has a preconceived model of what arthritis is from his teaching and past experience and the patient knows how he himself feels. The two views do not always coincide.

Do not be afraid to ask questions of your doctor. If you do not understand the answers, get your doctor to go over it again using different words until you are sure you understand.

If you have more than one or two questions it is a good idea to write them down, because it is very easy to get absorbed in a discussion on one point and forget your next question. If the doctor's answer is complicated with a number of points you have to remember such as, "Take one of the pink tablets before breakfast and two yellow ones at lunch time and three of the little white ones at night," write it down, or better still get the doctor to do so. Spot checks on patients coming out of doctors' surgeries reveal that patients actually remember very little of what doctors tell them and regularly misunderstand dosage schedules.

If the doctor advises exercise, make certain you understand how much and in what form he intends you to take it. Exercise means different things to different people, ranging from a fast sprint to gentle stretching and contracting of specific muscles. Make sure you know which.

Do not be afraid to ask the meaning of medical jargon words. Doctors talk their own language to one another because it is accurate and quick. Sometimes they forget when talking to patients that they are using words which may be unfamiliar.

Sometimes doctors give advice which at first sight does not seem related to the problem, such as telling a patient with pain in the hips to lose weight. If you do not see the point of such advice, ask why, and the doctor will then explain that every added pound puts extra strain on the joint.

If you find that the advice your doctor gives you is impossible to follow, say so. The doctor will often be able to find another way of achieving the same result but he cannot read your mind, and unless you put up an objection he will take your silence for agreement.

Ask the main question on your mind early in the consultation even if it seems silly or embarrassing. Nothing is more likely to irritate the doctor than to spend time talking about unimportant trivia and, just when the consultation is being wound up, to say, "While I am here, doctor," and then come out with the real reason for your visit.

If your doctor will not answer questions or discuss your problems, you may want to think about finding another doctor.

In short, to get the best from your doctor, be a C.A.D.

Come prepared   Ask questions   Discuss problems

A doctor's addendum: I have never seen a person with arthritis whom I could not help. There are some individuals, however, whom I have not helped. In every such case, the communication broke down. Sometimes I am short of time or short of temper. Sometimes the person doesn't listen or doesn't hear or doesn't understand. Often a preconceived opinion is the problem. "Aspirin won't work." "My neighbour couldn't tolerate that drug." "I hardly eat a thing." "She seems too old to exercise." "I don't think he would understand." Or a person who reports being worse never had the prescription made up, stopped an exercise programme after two days, decreased medication ("It made me too sleepy") and never mentioned the problem. A solid half of the blame lies with the doctor. Sometimes we do not listen or have our own preconceived ideas. No matter how hard we try we don't always get it right. But the other half of the blame lies with the patient. Tell it true and straight and we can help. This is a partnership. We don't always have to agree to get good results. But the give and take of direct communication is essential.

HELPFUL ORGANIZATIONS

Arthritis Care
6 Grosvenor Crescent, London SW1X 7ER
Tel. 01-235 0902/5
Arthritis Care is a welfare organization which provides information, advice and practical aid to arthritis and rheumatism sufferers. It has branches throughout the country and membership is open to all sufferers, also to anyone interested in giving financial or active help. There is a very modest annual subscription. It serves to keep arthritis sufferers in contact with each other, which can be a great morale booster to the socially isolated, provides holiday accommodation and runs a welfare department to give advice on all aspects of the day-to-day living problems of arthritis sufferers. It publishes *Arthritis News*, a regular paper which keeps members in touch with the Association's activities and has cookery, gardening and other features of special interest to disabled people, and contributions from distinguished writers. Membership of Arthritis Care is strongly recommended to all sufferers.

The Arthritis and Rheumatism Council for Research
41 Eagle Street, London WC1R 4AR
Tel. 01-405 8572
The Council acts to co-ordinate research into all aspects of arthritis and
rheumatic diseases. It promotes academic positions in rheumatology at
universities and facilitates the training of junior doctors in rheumatology.
Much work has been done under its auspices into the epidemiology of
rheumatism, which helps doctors to understand how rheumatism develops
in the individual and how the condition affects the community as a whole.
It serves to spread knowledge of developments in treatment to the medical
profession and widens the provision of specialist treatment. it publishes
ARC (3 issues per year) magazine for all those involved in the development
of rheumatology. It also publishes a number of useful handbooks for patients.

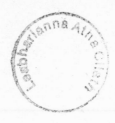

BIBLIOGRAPHY

1   Handbooks for patients published by the Arthritis and Rheumatism
    Council for Research, 41 Eagle Street, London WC1 4AR.
    Free pamphlets on specific conditions
    Rheumatoid Arthritis
    Osteoarthritis
    Ambylosis Spondylitis
    Gout
    Pain in the Neck
    Lumbar Disc Disorders
    General handbooks
    A Guide to Arthritis and Other Rheumatic Diseases
    Your Home and Your Rheumatism
    Marriage, Sex and Arthritis
    When Your Child Has Arthritis
2   Books published by the Disabled Living Foundation, 346 Kensington
    High Street, London W14
    Coping with Disablement, edited by Peggy Jay, 3rd edition 1983.

Kitchen Sense for Disabled or Elderly People, edited by Sydney Foott, revised reprint 1976.

Clothes Sense for Handicapped Adults of All Ages, by P. Macartney, 1973.

Dressing for Disabled People, by Rosemary Ruston, revised edition 1982.

The Easy Path to Gardening, 1972 (in association with the Readers Digest Association).

3   *Rheumatism and Arthritis*, by Malcolm I. V. Jayson & Allan St.J. Dixon, 1974, Pan Books, London.

4   *Understanding Rheumatism*, by F. Dudley Hart, revised edition 1982, Family Doctor Publications, BMA House, Tavistock Square, London WC2.

5   *Overcoming Arthritis*, by F. Dudley Hart, 1981, Martin Dunitz Ltd., London, available from Mitchell Beazley Ltd., Artist House, 14 Manette Street, London W1.

6   *Handling the Handicapped*, a guide to the lifting and movement of disabled people, 2nd edition 1980, The Chartered Society of Physiotherapy in association with Woodhead Faulkner Ltd., 17 Market Street, Cambridge CB2 3PA.

7   *Directory for the Disabled*, edited by Ann Darnbrough & Derek Kinrade, 3rd edition 1982, Woodhead Faulkner Ltd., 17 Market Street, Cambridge CB2 3PA.

8   *Home Made Aids for Handicapped People*, revised edition 1974, the British Red Cross Society, available from the Society's shop at 4 Grosvenor Crescent, London SW1.

9   *Diet for Life*, by Mary Laver & Margaret Smith, 1981, Pan Books, London.

10 *Handicapped Living*, a monthly magazine available from leading newsagents or from the publishers, Living Publications Ltd., 9 West Street, Epsom, Surrey, KT18 7RL.

Index